BOLDY
BALD
WOMEN

PAM FITROS

©2013
Nightengale Press
A Nightengale Media LLC Company

BOLDLY BALD WOMEN

For information about Nightengale Press please
visit our website at www.nightengalepress.com.
Email: publisher@nightengalepress.com
or send a letter to:
Nightengale Press
370 S. Lowe Avenue, Suite A-122
Cookeville, Tennessee

Library of Congress Cataloging-in-Publication Data

Fitros Pam,

BOLDLY BALD WOMEN/ Pam Fitros

ISBN 13: 978-1-935993-41-4
Health & Wellness, Non-fiction

Copyright Registered: 2013
First Published by Nightengale Press in the USA

January 2013

10 9 8 7 6 5 4 3 2 1

Printed in the USA and the UK

KUDOS

Pam Fitros has found a life calling to educate others about hair loss, whether through the curious looks of a child in the grocery store or on these pages. Her words are as warm as a personal letter just for you. She will love you into understanding the challenges of women with alopecia.

Pam Fitros says, "My baldness is what I have that makes me different." This isn't the only thing which sets Pam apart from others. Her tenaciously coated, loving heart spills out on these pages to inform, entertain and encourage. Boldly Bald Women will help anyone facing the challenges of hair loss find courage to face and alleviate personal fears and find they are not alone on this journey. Carry-on Ladies... with confidence, personal fortitude, guts and persistence.

As a woman of hair who complains about and uses bad hair days as an excuse... I now have a new definition of courage: "to unwrap ones head of all disguises and walk boldly into the world." Now I'm wondering, is my hair holding me back?

—Ellen Peterson, blog author of When all is said and done... I'll still have something to say! http://ellepeterson.wordpress.com/

☞☜

Pam Fitros expertly and proudly puts the 'bold' into Boldly Bald. By sharing her own and others' stories with fire and courage, her book emerges as an inspiration to women who either can't, or won't, wear wigs to cover their bald heads. You go, girl!"

—Leslie Ann Butler, Author of the nationally award-winning book, "If Your Hair Falls Out, Keep Dancing!"

☞☜

THIS is the book I needed to read when I was first diagnosed with alopecia areata! THIS is the book I wish I'd had when I was struggling with going out in public bald. Highly recommended for anyone at any stage of hair loss, or for people with an Alopecian in your life.

—Mary Marshall, Creator of "International Alopecia Day"™

෪ඏ

Reading to put your anxieties to sleep for long winter's night.
—Mike Larson, Photographer

෪ඏ

"*Whether you are bald by choice or by nature you need to read this book. You will share the joy and pain of those who have contributed to this work. More than that, you will feel comfort in their company - you will never be alone again. If I wasn't already bald, I would want to shave my head after reading this....*"
—shine on sista, Joyce Brier, Artist, Jewelry Designer

෪ඏ

"*Pam Fitros brings her own brand of humor and understanding to a sometimes challenging situation. Being a woman who is both a cancer survivor and totally bald due to alopecia, Pam shares her personal experiences along with the experiences of others who have been affected by hair loss. Boldly Bald Women, is an inspiring read for all bald women and their families, friends, co-workers and physicians.*"
—Sandy and Olivia Rusk, Olivia's Cause, www.oliviascause.org

෪ඏ

"*I lost my hair over twenty years ago, when it was just about unheard of for a woman to go without a wig. Most of my journey to embracing my life as a bald woman was made alone. The message in this book definitely would have made my journey easier. I am confident it will do just that for others.*"
—Cheryl Carvery-Jones, co-founder of AlopeciaWorld.com

෪ඏ

Dedication

To all women everywhere who struggle
with the emotional and social impacts of hair loss.

acknowledgements

When I began writing Boldly Bald Women I believed writing to be a solitary endeavor. I couldn't have been more wrong. Without a solid support system, there can be no sustained writing. Without a nudge along the way, it is easy to get waylaid and sidetracked. I understand that now, and I know who I need to acknowledge and why.

First, my mother, who told me I was a good writer so many times from childhood on that writing became ingrained into my core identity.

Thanks to Mike Larson for picking up my mother's mantra and encouraging me year after year with, "Are you writing? Why not?" And for all of his patience, photos and shared laughter.

I am grateful both to ovarian cancer and alopecia for giving me something I could write about from my heart.

Thank you, Pam Wardell, for doing without our Wednesday lunches so many times when the muse was whispering, and I knew the thought would be gone if I interrupted it.

There was a point where I was ready to walk away from this project. Valerie Connelly, my savvy publisher and now dear friend, sent me an email that verbally kicked me around the block. She refused to let me out of my contract because I was "discounting my ability as a writer, discounting the value of the book, and discounting her ability as an editor and publisher."

My sister, Diane, cheered when I read her the email, and said she'd decided to build Valerie a monument. After a short silence during which she blinked several times while deep in thought, she said, "I don't know how to build monuments. I'll make Valerie an afghan—the most beautiful afghan she will ever see. But she doesn't get it until I have a printed book in my hands." She made the afghan.

It is beyond exquisite. Diane would work on the afghan when we were together, lift an eyebrow casually and ask, "How many words did you write today? You know, Valerie doesn't get this until you finish." It worked. Without these two women, I would have abandoned Boldly Bald Women.

I thank my brother, David, whose gift enabled me to finance the cost involved in publishing Boldly Bald Women. I miss him every day. I know he would have been pleased with how his gift was used.

Thank you, Joyce Sherman Brier, for the fun of going to the NAAF conference together, for the many phone calls, the empathy, all the love, and the wonderful jewelry designs. You are a rock of can-do.

Thank you, Mary Marshall, for untold support, technical assistance and advice, for your belief in the value of Boldly Bald Women, and your determination to get it into the hands of everyone who may benefit from it.

Thank you Cheryl Carvery Jones for Alopecia World. Without it and the women I met there Boldly Bald Women would not exist.

I thank the women who shared their stories, giving so much time and energy to enlighten and encourage our bald and balding sisters, and our sisters' families, friends, physicians, employers and coworkers. They are the heart of Boldly Bald Women. All along the way they have given me encouragement and fortitude. You can see them in the photos at the end of the book.

And now, Hrisostomos Fitros, aka, Mike, the little Greek, and, Hey, Greek—my husband, my love, my best friend, and supporter of my desire to mark this book off my Bucket List. Thank you most of all. You have washed dishes, made dinners, helped with household chores, and fallen asleep on the couch way too many nights while watching TV by yourself without grumbling—much—as I tapped away on the computer keyboard into the night. Thank you, Mike, so very much, I recognize your actions as a gift of truest love. I love you too, my dear Greek, more with each passing year.

Yes, writing is not a solitary endeavor. Thank you. Thank you all. Thank you for your belief in me and your belief that this book can help hurting women find their way to self acceptance and courage and the emotional freedom to be Boldly Bald Women should they so choose.

—Pam Fitros

THIS THING CALLED ALOPECIA
by Dotty Jenkins

Okay, world, where do I start?
I guess I'll tell it from the heart.
It all began seven years ago,
Why it picked me, I still don't know.

It may be heredity, it may be stress,
All I knew was the doctor's guess.
There is no cause, no known cure,
You'll lose more hair, that's for sure.

You may lose some or lose it all,
No way to know how much will fall.
This can't be true! This isn't fair!
I'm a woman! I need my hair!

This thing called Alopecia, didn't stall,
Within three months I lost it all.
No scalp hair, brows or lashes now,
I had to accept the loss—but how?

I felt alone, I couldn't share,
I just cried, I didn't care.
I bought some wigs, they hid it well,
My Alopecia? None could tell.

Tried everything my doctor suggested,
Still all my hair, my body rejected.
Three years later I had no hair,
Three years living with despair.

One fine day I went online,
Where I met new friends of mine.
Alopecia groups, how nice,
I go to them for advice.

Alopecia won't discriminate
From age one to ninety-eight.
Not caring who or where you are,
In the USA or from afar.

If you're black or white or red,
It takes your hair right off your head.
Hair may come back or maybe not,
Is there anything else I forgot?

Yes! Alopecians, beautiful inside and out,
We need to show what that's about.
Alopecians, neither freaks nor contagious,
Thinking otherwise is outrageous.

I lost all my hair, not my identity,
My Alopecian friends give me serenity.
So, give us a chance and don't make fun,
Alopecians are just like everyone!

FOREWORD

Never believe that a few caring people can't change the world. For, indeed, that's all who ever have.
—Margaret Mead

⪶⪵

Meet yourself with love wherever you are in the process of hair loss, whatever the reason for your hair loss.

⪶⪵

Treat yourself as kindly as you would someone else going through a time of loss and identity change, knowing how painful being different can be.

⪶⪵

Gather information with the understanding you don't ever have to go bald into the world, if you choose not to.

⪶⪵

Reach out to the available support around you and join a community of those who understand.

⪶⪵

Believe in your own God-given value and beauty and let go of all self doubt and deprecation to enable others to see that value and beauty in its true form.

⪶⪵

Know that you have the power within you to contribute to a tomorrow that enthusiastically welcomes and embraces Boldly Bald Women.

⪶⪵

BOLDLY BALD women

CHAPTER 1

Alopecia—It's a Real Trip

᷅᷄

Life is a journey through time.
Happiness is what happens when we take that journey together.
—Dr. Daniel Gilbert

᷅᷄

I was a short-haired girl most of my adult life, and I considered hair a nuisance. I got crabby when it was time for a haircut and my bangs hung in front of my eyes. Oh, sure, hair could be attractive, but what about all those other times? You know—when you wake up in the morning with chicken-butt hair all at odds and angles? When your hair outgrows your bottled color and the shadow of your smile is eclipsed by shadow of your roots? What about all the time and money spent for cuts and coloring and perms and straightening? There is a line of must-have products as long as the imaginations of hair care gurus—whose biggest delight is to part women from their money.

And it doesn't stop there. No. Then comes the eyebrow shaping, the nose hair trimming, the mustache waxing, and the tweezing of those long, coarse goat-beard-middle-aged-chin-hairs!

I imagined it would be great to be like Yule Brenner, or Telly Savalis, or Mr. Clean. Such freedom! They had no hair on their heads and yet were considered exotic and sexy. Why couldn't it be that way for women too? Science fiction gave us some bald females, but you had to be a Star Trek alien to be bald and exotic and sexy. Baldness in real women in the real world is associated with illness, undesirability, and shame.

The hardest part of losing hair to alopecia universalis—for most women—is the feeling of utter isolation resulting from that hair loss. Up until recently, everything from bald spots to bald heads have been covered up, and not spoken about above a whisper.

Cancer patients on chemotherapy expect to lose their hair. They are prepared by their physicians for the possibility, if not the probability, of total hair loss. In some hospitals, chemo is done in a group setting. Women go through the process together. They get to know each other and gain courage and strength from each other. They bring knitting and crocheting and share patterns and techniques or read books to each other to wile away the time. They count treatments left to do and crack jokes to keep each other going. They grieve the loss of a friend whenever death intervenes in recovery. I know this because I was in and out of the cancer center often enough to observe the bonding process.

In 2005, I was diagnosed with ovarian cancer. It turned out that instead of normal walnut sized ovaries, one of my ovaries was the size of a lemon. The other had grown to the size of a melon. Both were full of cancer. Seventy-five percent of women diagnosed with ovarian cancer die from it. I joked that between chemo and radiation I'd surely turn into Mrs. Clean, free of chicken-butt hair at last. But it was not to be. After a total hysterectomy, my gynecological oncologist, the most excellent doctor, Kevin Brader, at the Lacks Cancer Center in Grand Rapids, Michigan, announced he'd gotten everything without puncturing the ovaries. Nothing had metastasized to any other parts of my body. I was spared both chemo and radiation therapies. Thank you, Dr. Brader. You are both an incredibly skilled surgeon and the most tender-hearted of men.

Some might call me fortunate. I call myself blessed. I am blessed to have been led to an outstanding doctor, blessed to have had such a miraculous outcome. Obviously Poppa God is not done with me yet. Still, be careful what you wish for, even in jest, because you might just get it.

Three years later, I had a reaction to severe stress that apparently triggered an autoimmune response. The result was alopecia universalis. My hyper-vigilant immune system was trying to protect me. It decided my hair must be an invading enemy, and so, attacked the hair follicles of my body.

Patch by patch, here a clump, there a clump, everywhere a clump, clump, arm hair, nose hair, ear hair, every hair. The process was not as cool as I'd imagined the result would be. Except for the shedding of those ridiculous chin hairs, it's not a lot of fun to gather hair from your pillow every morning and clean out the clogged drain with every shower. How I wished for the kind of mutual support I had seen in Lacks Cancer Center as I lost every hair on my body to alopecia over a two-month period. How I wished I had known even one other woman with alopecia.

I'd made a date with a girlfriend for lunch and a movie. When she saw me, she wrapped her arms around me and said, "Pammy, we're not going to lunch and a movie, we're going to lunch and a wig shop. You know I love you no matter what, but I've seen dogs with mange that look better than you do."

We both laughed uproariously. If anyone else told me I looked worse than a dog with mange, I would have been mortified and terribly hurt. From that dear friend, it was a gift of acceptance and a call to action. I no longer had to sit passively and do nothing but anxiously pretend the silver dollar sized patches didn't show. After lunch, and fortified by splitting a piece of Snicker's ice cream pie, we trundled off to the wig shop. We both had a blast trying on wigs of all colors, lengths, and styles.

Not one to dither when I've found a direction that feels right, I had the rest of my hair buzzed and went home wearing my new wig. Some people thought I'd had my hair colored and styled. Some didn't notice anything. Some said I looked ten years younger. It was fun, for a few days, until I started getting headaches from maintaining a tight enough fit to keep the wig on. I watched penciled eyebrows slide down my cheeks in rivulets of sweat from my overheated head. Recurring yeast infections on my scalp were literally the icing on the cupcake of baldness. I was miserable.

When you have alopecia you can't exactly walk up to a cancer patient and say: "Woe is me, I've lost my hair!" They are in a battle for their lives. Hair loss is devastating for cancer victims too, sometimes more emotionally devastating than the cancer itself, but hair loss is not the primary focus. Beating cancer is the primary focus. Besides, hair will usually grow back when treatments stop. Sometimes straight when it was curly or curly if it was straight, sometimes a different color, but it usually grows back. Alopecia universalis, the most extreme of the alopecias, is, in its extremity, most often a permanent condition.

When I lost my hair I was physically healthy, well, at least I was as healthy as an overweight, middle-aged woman with allergies, arthritic knees, high cholesterol, and borderline diabetes can be. It turns out that a lot of women with alopecia have similar conditions.

I began to understand. Yes, wearing a wig took care of the outside problem, if you didn't count melting makeup. But inside, a wig-wearing bald woman doesn't ever get to forget she's bald. The sense of unconscious self is erased. Inside, part of you is always aware, always on alert for clues that might suddenly give you away.

Casual physical contact became constrained for me. Is my hair on straight? Hugs became mine fields of sagging and snagging potential. Anxiety over the condition, position, and stability of my fake hair took predominance in my thoughts. And I got angry—very, very angry that men could choose to deal with a balding condition by shaving their heads, shining them up and sauntering into the world to be viewed as sophisticated and virile, while bald women felt it necessary to hide to be presentable and sexy.

I love hugs. I love giving them and receiving them. I love hugs as an expression of caring and connection. I love them as reassurance and encouragement. I love hugs as greetings and goodbyes, as the exclamation points of joy and excitement and the absorptive tissues of sorrow. It is said we need four hugs per day for survival; eight per day for maintenance, and twelve hugs a day for growth. I was definitely in growth mode.

But when I lost my hair and donned that wig, my hugs turned wiggy too. The slang term of wiggy is "excited, eccentric, crazy." The rarer usage of wiggy is "pompously formal." When I wore that wig, hugs became both crazy and took on an uncomfortable formality. Was the person I was hugging wearing glasses or anything on their ears that might get caught in the fibers of my wig? Did their clothing pose any threat? What danger lay in wait from a benign piece of jewelry? Was my overheated head dripping sweat? It took a high degree of concentration to navigate the obstacle course to give or get a hug.

If someone came up behind me while I was sitting in a chair, looking up and back over my shoulder to see who it was, pushed the wig up higher on my scalp. It formed a large mound on top of my head as though I'd magically transformed my hairdo into the teased bubble style of the Sixties. Worse yet, it would start to slip off sideways, and I'd smack the top of my head to ram it back into place. You can imagine how professional that looked. Not!

I became hyper-vigilant and protective of my movements. I worked at a retirement home and worried that a bald head might be offensive to, or stressful for, the residents. My hugs became stiff and formal. It was a really bad case of wiggy hugs. I resented the loss of my spontaneity. People asked: "What's happened to you? Are you all right?"

"Nooo!" I finally wailed one day. "I'm not all right. I've lost my hair and I'm wearing a wig and the stupid thing gets caught on everything and drags around sideways on my head. I constantly have to check if it's on straight. I'm sweating like a pig and I'm getting very hug-deprived and crabby—it's driving me crazy."

After a moment of startled silence, one resident shuffled up to me with her walker and whispered into my ear, "Then take the damn thing off!" She was very hard of hearing and didn't realize her whisper-volume was permanently stuck on LOUD. I looked around. The rest of the women were sagely nodding their heads in agreement.

It occurred to me that the people I was most worried about offending were the very ones who'd rather have real hugs than fake hair. When I got home that night, I took the wig off. That was the beginning of a journey into a whole new world of both introspection and outreach that has led me to a place of genuine gratitude for alopecia universalis. It is not unusual for friends and family to see me doing the Snoopy happy dance, if not with my whole body, at least with the sparkle in my eyes which is now only enhanced by the shine of my boldly bald head.

Whether you are a bald woman, or someone who knows or loves a bald woman or child, I invite you to share this journey with me. It has become much greater and more exciting than I ever imagined. There are challenges ahead and stories and laughter and tears, and a newly found network of amazing support and camaraderie.

Most of all this is a journey to understanding, acceptance, and hope for those women who, for what ever reason, got off the Life Train at the same station I did: Bald Boulevard. If you've picked up this book you've already paid for your ticket. All aboard!

CHAPTER 2
You're Not Alone

⧃⧂

Women are never stronger
than when they arm themselves with their weakness.
—Marie de Vichy-Chamrond, Marquise de Deffand, 1697-1780

⧃⧂

"You're not alone ."
"Yah, sure!"
"No, really, you're not alone."

If you are new to alopecia—to hair loss from any reason—it is common to feel alone and want to hide. We all have a self-image that is drastically altered by hair loss. It takes time to grieve that loss and adjust to the new reflection in the mirror. During that time we are especially vulnerable to the furtive glances and comments family and friends make in reaction to our changed appearance, as well those of strangers who gawk and whisper or point and *inform* us we have no hair.

How can we hope to cope with the reactions of others when we look in the mirror to see a startle reaction at our own reflection and weep for the strange woman looking woefully back?

I asked women with adult onset alopecia to write about their

BOLDLY BALD WOMEN

initial reaction to hair loss. Perhaps you'll find an echo of your own feelings in one of theirs.

❖ *Panic. My hair was my signature, what I was well-known for in my social circle. My shoulder length, bone straight, healthy flowing hair. I didn't cry—I hate crying.*

—Galena

❖ *I was mortified that I was losing hair in huge clumps. I was in a new relationship and thought I was hiding it well, but it got to be so much loss that I needed to fess up about what was going on.*

—Carol S.

❖ *Shocked, surprised, confused, frantic. I wasn't kind to myself, got into bad company and became dependent on drink and drugs. I hid away and moped around.*

—Sharon

❖ *Waking up every morning with a pillow full of hair and seeing half of my hair in the drain every time I took a shower was too much for me to take. I was even afraid to brush or comb my hair for fear of pulling the rest out!*

—Dotty

❖ *Devastation. I was traumatized. Of course, the more I worried, the worse it became. I have a twin sister, and I am ashamed to say that I felt bitter that this was happening to me. I also suffer with severe eczema and asthma and so with this, on top of all that, I felt unable to cope. I became very low and all my confidence was knocked out of me.*

—Gwennan

❖ *I was HORRIFIED! I was sure that I was dying at first. And sadly, my primary care physician didn't tell me otherwise.*

—Sandy

23

BOLDLY BaLD Women

❖ *Completely freaked out. I was just twenty-five years old. Yet, I was relieved I wasn't diagnosed with a terminal disease of any kind. Alopecia Areata has a ring of 'cure' to its name, I thought. Boy, was I wrong. I was in denial and avoided mirrors and just hoped no one would notice.*

—*Kristine*

❖ *Surprise, but not too much anxiety because the spots were small, infrequent and not visible. Later, when it progressed rapidly, I became very depressed, cried a lot and constantly checked my head for expansion of the bald areas.*

—*Mary*

The same holds true for children with alopecia. Parents ask, "How could this be happening to *our* child? What can we do to protect her? How can we help him cope? Where can we get help?"

Here are some of the responses from women with childhood onset of alopecia:

❖ Jo, a second generation holocaust survivor began, losing her hair at fourteen. Her Dutch family immigrated to Australia after over eighty of her extended family members were exterminated in the WWII death camps. Jo, a small, delicate child, suffered from numerous allergies, asthma, and eczema and had experienced much bullying and teasing for her differences early in life. She says: *"Looking different due to eczema and alopecia made me a target. People were afraid I was contagious. I would sit alone, be ridiculed, laughed at, prodded and poked. My mother blamed me for using the hair dryer and didn't want to accept what the doctors told her—that it was immune related."*

BOLDLY BALD WOMEN

❖ *My name is Sarah. I'm now thirty-five years old, but my relationship with alopecia dates back many years to when I was just thirteen. I began losing hair in patches soon after I reached puberty. It was a stressful time in my life. I was being presented with many challenging issues. Some had to do with my family and others included what might be considered the usual teenage confusion and angst. I was definitely feeling strain. I remember quite vividly the very day my hair started falling out, or at least when I first noticed it. My family and I were on a drive back home from a short trip to Chicago. I ran my fingers through my hair, which was long and blonde, and came away with a fistful. I was absolutely shocked and horrified.*

Over the next days and weeks, I noticed a lot more hair falling out, mostly because in the morning I would awaken to a small pile of it on my pillow, and then again in the shower when the drain plug was covered in unusual amounts of hair. It started becoming very visibly noticeable, and soon some of the kids at school were making rude comments and teasing me. I didn't know what was happening or why and neither did my family.

If I hadn't been really stressed out before my hair started falling out, I sure was now. Soon, I was no longer able to bring myself to go to school. It changed the way I looked at the world and the way I saw myself. Prior to my hair falling out I was a fairly attractive, popular young teen. I was, like so many others my age, very caught up in superficial appearances. When my hair fell out, I was suddenly thrust into a new awareness. I had always been a fairly sensitive and somewhat introverted person, and losing my hair to alopecia caused me to go further inward. People in general can be very unkind about looking different, and teenagers can be downright cruel. A couple of my nicknames were Kojak and

25

BOLDLY BALD WOMEN

Mr. Clean, not exactly what a fourteen-year-old girl aspires to be compared to.

I was laughed at, taunted, heckled and even physically threatened at different times. Once, when I was walking down a city street with a male friend, he was jumped by a teenage group of African American males who had wrongly assumed I was a skinhead and decided to take it out on my friend. This event was particularly difficult for me to accept because my friend bore the brunt of it. When I moved to a new school and started 9th grade I was introduced to my first class and several of the students snickered and laughed out loud. It was utterly humiliating.

—Sarah

❖ *I've had alopecia since I was twelve. In the fall of seventh grade, I started losing my hair along the left side, and it gradually went around the back and up the other side. It was first discovered by my regular doctor during a follow-up for an ear infection. He noticed something funny about my hairline behind my ear and recommended I go to a dermatologist.*

I was scared and my immediate thought was: "I'm going to die." When the dermatologist put a name to this oddity on my scalp, I felt relieved. However, as my hair loss worsened, so did my self-confidence. I went into an angry, depressed state which I kept bottled up inside because I did not want my peers or any family, besides my parents, to know.

I think the age you are when you develop alopecia has a huge impact on your reaction and attitude towards it. Being twelve, when you're just kind of entering womanhood, you just started your period around that time and you're developing breasts and, you know, hormones, and you're interested in boys—I think it did some damage that I never really got past.

BOLDLY BALD WOMEN

I didn't want anyone to know. Well into high school, limited people knew. I would hide in the closet if someone came over unexpectedly, or pretend I was sleeping on the couch with the pillow over my head and wouldn't go outside without a wig. I didn't tell my two best friends in middle school for the first year. And even when I did, I just said (quickly), "I have alopecia and this makes me lose my hair." I didn't go into detail. I didn't want to talk about it or get upset in front of them. I was struggling and I didn't want to let on how much I was hurting. I didn't want to be a burden to them, so I just cried to my mom and dad.

I believe grief plays a role in your hair loss. I definitely grieved the hair that I had. You imagine your life to be a certain way and yourself to look a certain way in that vision and when you don't, it is life altering. Literally, you have to re-adjust how to see yourself and who you are. You have to grieve the death of what you thought could be.

—Caitlin

❖ *I lost my hair when I was seven years old. It seemed to have fallen out overnight. I remember my mother vacuuming my pillow as the hair came out in clumps. My parents didn't know what to do or which doctor to take me to. I guess they felt helpless. I was terrified with all that was happening within me and around me. I was left always feeling like I didn't belong. I would often retreat to my bedroom and cry. I would be outside making mud pies, and I would cry. It seemed all I did was cry.*

—Willow

❖ Olivia lost her hair when she was too young to have any response to alopecia, so her mother, Sandy, responded from her own perspective.

Olivia first experienced alopecia at eighteen months of age. Her hair loss was very rapid—within four weeks—but she only lost the hair on her head (alopecia totalis). We visited numerous doctors and tried several different topical treatments. We finally located Dr. Patricia Treadwell, the top pediatric dermatologist at Riley Children's Hospital. She prescribed a topical steroid (Clobetasol) and Women's Rogaine. It took about two years but about ninety-five percent of Olivia's hair did re-grow. However, four years later she lost all of it a second time. This time she lost all her body hair (alopecia universalis), too. All the doctors showed very little sympathy or support. They just stated that it was alopecia and that they did not know what caused it and that they did not know if or when it would re-grow. At the time, we did not have the Internet resources that we have today, and as a mom of a small child with this mysterious condition, I did not know where to turn. I was an emotional mess. My initial reaction to Olivia's alopecia was shock. I had never heard of this condition and could not believe that most of the doctors I met were of no help. As a single mom, I was handling it all on my own and was just devastated.

As with most of us, more than meets the eye was going on with some of these women and children. I have left out the more personal details of what was happening in their lives when hair loss began, because whatever the reason for the onset, it is the reactions to hair loss itself which I seek to illuminate. The admirable women in Boldly Bald Women share their stories of found courage and emotional strength candidly in the hope that something in their experiences might help someone reading *Boldly Bald Women*.

BOLDLY BALD WOMEN

Whether you're new to hair loss or have lived with baldness for years, remember this: you are not alone. Others know the depth of the grief and pain you feel now or have felt at some point in your journey. Others have awakened to clumps of hair on their pillow and soggy wet clogs of it in the shower. Others understand the fear of rejection, as well as, sometimes, the devastating reality of it. Others have reached deep within and found their courage, exercised their strength, and made a way for themselves. Some have floundered, hidden their heads out of shame and fear or from the necessities of cultural taboo.

When I asked Galena about finding acceptance for her alopecia, she responded:

I won't call it acceptance. I call it moving on and not inflicting self-pity and pain. I call it another issue like all of the other issues I face in my life. It is what it is. I'm an approachable person, but I really hate explaining my hair loss. I don't solicit responses from people and being a bald woman solicits responses from people, verbally, but mostly non-verbally.

About how alopecia has changed the way others have seen her, Galena says:

I don't know. I feel an energy that is admiration of my courage. I don't burden others and I candidly answer all enquires with a practiced grace and humor. Some, including my husband, say I look beautiful with or without hair. One gorgeous woman at church says I look sexy, and she appears to be sincere. I deeply appreciate the good energy. I don't take it for granted. I thank God that I was never conceited or people would not be so kind at this time.

I asked Galena how coping with alopecia changed the way she saw herself.

Acceptance of alopecia is the result of going through a dark place.

BOLDLY BALD WOMEN

That might seem overly dramatic, but it's not just about my appearance—there has been a complete transformation. I liken it to the myth of the Phoenix burning away and arising from the ashes. There is a reason for this and, while I'm on this journey of being an Alopecian, I will love myself and learn all that I'm supposed to. There are no dress rehearsals in life.

Whoever you are, wherever you are, whether the hair loss is yours or that of someone you care about and aren't sure how to help, you are not alone. You are in good company—the best of company.

CHAPTER 3
Quit Whining Kermit—Green Is Easy

❧❧

What lies behind us and what lies before us are tiny matters compared to what lies within us.
—Ralph Waldo Emerson

❧❧

Kermit the Frog, of Jim Henson's Muppet fame, fusses over how hard he thinks it is to be green. Bald didn't faze him at all. But then, Kermit is a boy Muppet. Miss Piggy, also naturally bald, co-quettishly flicks the long blond wig which is as much a part of her signature persona as her strident high pitched voice.

So, why IS it such a big deal for women, even Muppet women, to choose to be boldly bald?

Hair is a visual language. It gives us up to the minute information about others. The language of hair, like all languages, morphs through time and cultures, but in every time and in every culture, hair broadcasts the condition, social standing and, in some societies, even the marital status of women. Hence, a glance at a woman's hair supposedly signals the degree of her attractiveness and availability.

My brother married when I was sixteen. I was in the wedding. That was in the '60s when the bubble style was popular. I wanted the chestnut locks of my hair to be perfect for my brother's wedding.

BOLDLY BALD WOMEN

So I carefully teased and styled until the perfected hair do was just right. Then I worried about keeping it in place for the duration of the wedding. So I sprayed it with hair spray. I let that dry and sprayed it again. And then once more just to be sure.

As nervous, excited bridesmaids and self-conscious groomsmen lined up to start down the church aisle, the fellow to walk with me stared at my hair. I was sure I'd missed a spot and something was out of place. Panic swirled in the angst of my teenage mind. The young man said: "Excuse me; I just have to touch your hair." He poked his index finger at the side of my head and looked startled. Nothing had moved. His touch hadn't made a dent in my lacquered do. "It's like a helmet," he whispered, eyes wide in amazement.

I sighed, relieved. It would hold up, I affirmed. Who knew I would end up being one of the reasons the bubble-do would become famous as helmet hair! That was back in the days when sixteen-year-old girls were a lot younger and more naïve than sixteen-year-olds of today. It took a couple of hours to figure out the guy's response was not a compliment.

In the language of hair, the meaning of bald has been simple and clear: stay away; unhealthy; repulsive. Who wants to be a walking advertisement for ugly? I, for one, do not. Up until now, the only acceptable option available for bald women has been hiding their baldness.

Some of us have had more than enough of hiding. Women are beginning to pioneer a new option, boldly bald. It's time for the language of hair to evolve to include some new meanings for female baldness. Who better to define those meanings than the women who, every day, face the anxiety and shame baldness imparts, all the while knowing they are just as healthy, intelligent and sexy, without hair as they ever were with hair.

BOLDLY BALD WOMEN

Let's start by making one very important clarification right up front. Boldly Bald Women are not just as; they are more than. Living openly with alopecia requires courage and stamina and humor...all of which are great character builders. I haven't met one woman living openly with baldness who hasn't developed a delightful depth of character that glows and sparkles with her ability to make delicious lemonade of life's lemons. Not many of us would have chosen bald deliberately, especially in view of how difficult it is to be bald in a society infatuated with women's hair. But those of us who have decided to live openly with the baldness our body has foisted upon us know a wealth of delightful freedom.

To move beyond the current definitions of beauty in the language of hair and make way for a new perspective on Boldly Bald, let's take a closer look at what those definitions are and how they came into being.

Two things became apparent as I researched the history of hair. One, public female baldness has historically never been looked upon as acceptable, let alone positive. Two, the history of women's hair is so tightly woven into the legal/social/political status of women that the history of hair has less to do with hair itself than with a woman's right to her own personhood.

An Historical Perspective

The distaste and shame associated with female baldness is rooted deeply in the history of the female gender. And, sorry guys, but the truth is the truth. Male dominated society planted that distaste and shame, grew it and then legislated and governed it, while the same men carved out rationales for their own baldness as being a result of superior intelligence and sexual virility.

Valerie Connelly, publisher of *Boldly Bald Women*, shared a story about her grandmother while we were editing this chapter. I share it with you now as an excellent example of male domination over women and their hair. Valerie's grandmother, Mary Cranston Green, was born in 1865, the year of Lincoln's assassination. She was the first woman to be enrolled into a small religious college in southern Illinois during the mid-1880's. She was to graduate with honors – a very, very big deal for a woman of that day and age.

Just before graduation day she cut her waist length hair into a just below the ears 'bob'. The president of the college was appalled. He told her in no uncertain terms he didn't think he could graduate her since she had shown such poor judgment in cutting her hair.

She drew herself up to full height, squared her shoulders and told the president politely, but with unshakable conviction, that the length of her hair had nothing to do with the quality and value of her mind. This plucky young woman not only graduated, but graduated with every honor she was due—except one. She should have gotten an additional honor for standing-up to that *educated* ignorant jerk. Okay, back to ancient history.

The Egyptians

There was, however, a shining moment for baldness about 5,400 years ago, beginning 3400 BC in Egypt—Camelot for the Boldly Bald, if you will. Egyptians, men, women, and children alike, shaved their hair off, both to avoid infestation of rampant head lice and for relief from an extremely hot climate.

The deliberate baldness of personal comfort, however, was not meant for public display. Hair was still important to convey visual messages of wealth, status and political significance. Not to mention protection from the harsh Egyptian sun. The wealthy had collections of expensive human hair wigs, culled from the hair of slaves. These were elaborately arranged and adorned with gem-encrusted, gold diadems, exquisitely carved hairpins of ivory, precious metals and beads—think Elizabeth Taylor in Cleopatra. The longest, most complicated styles were reserved for the highest class women. Those with less status and money used real hair extensions or combinations of plant fiber and hair. The bottom of the social heap wore wigs too, but they were made completely from vegetable fibers.

Wigs were status symbols to be sure, but they weren't meant to hide baldness in the same way the curtain in the chamber of the Wizard of Oz was meant to hide the lowly, symbolically powerless man behind the scenes. Wigs were items of fashion and fun and everybody knew everybody else was bald underneath them. At that time in history baldness held no dark connotations of ill health or shameful misdeeds.

Unlike most other ancient societies, women and men were equal under the law and viewed each other as equals. Men weren't in charge of an Egyptian woman's personal power and perceived value. Women of Egypt could own, manage and sell property. They could own and free slaves at will, make and sign contracts, make adoptions, and they were entitled to sue at law. Egyptian women didn't need a husband for economic security. And, once married they retained their rights. They could come and go as they pleased and divorce if they so chose.

The differences in people's legal rights came from their places in the pecking order of social class rather than from their gender, but, within each class there was equality between men and women. The life of lower class Egyptians was harsh. And, slaves were still slaves regardless of gender equality within their low social standing. Still, if I had to pick an era and place to be a bald woman other than in the here and now, it would have been Egypt in 3400 BC.

Beware of Greeks Bearing Gifts—Especially Intellectual Theories

Before we go any further, I must tell you I am married to a

BOLDLY BALD WOMEN

Greek man. He's adorable. He's wonderful. He's amazing. Short, but really amazing. He's my best friend, the love of my life. He makes me laugh every day and has promised me if I ever even think about writing another book, he'll cheerfully divorce me (he doesn't know it yet, but he doesn't mean that). Well, you get the picture. I have no animosity towards Greeks per se—except for two: Plato and Aristotle. I have a bone to pick with those boys.

It is the best for all tame animals to be ruled by human beings. For this is how they are kept alive. In the same way, the relationship between the male and the female is by nature such that the male is higher, the female lower, that the male rules and the female is ruled. (Aristotle, Politica, ed. Loeb Classical Library, 1254 b 10-14.)

People respected what Aristotle said. His impact on thoughts and beliefs was widespread and long lasting.

Plato, Aristotle's mentor, taught Aristotle that females were biologically inferior to males because they did not produce semen. Plato contended the soul of a human being was contained in the semen and women only supplied the nourishment, or medium, in which the form grew. The man was the seed; the woman was merely the field. Aristotle concluded that a woman's inability to produce semen was her deficiency and made her sub-human.

Sisters and brothers: that statement makes my feminist blood boil. This put Greek women—and all women from that time forward—in the position of being subjected to men in everything and legally powerless to alter their position. In some places women weren't even allowed to cut their own hair without a man's permission. Marriages were arranged along status lines to produce heirs for property inheritance. A woman's feelings weren't considered. She was looked upon as breeding stock. Her success in obtaining the financial stabil-

36

BOLDLY BALD WOMEN

ity of a husband was dependent on being perceived as valuable breeding stock *as defined by men*.

If time travel were a reality and if I were transported back to ancient Greece, I wouldn't have lasted very long. Once, in the early part of our relationship, my husband had some of his Greek buddies over to celebrate his name day (Greeks celebrate the calendar 'day' of the Saints they were named for rather than their birthdays. Everybody is named after some saint, or given to a saint who is the catch all for those not named after a particular saint.) When one of the fellows finished his beer, Mike asked if he'd like another. His friend, Gus, who came to the United States many years before, nodded. Mike snapped his fingers, gesturing for me to bring another beer. Gus cringed and gasped.

"What?" Mike asked in a bewildered tone.

"Never, never snap your fingers at an American woman," Gus whispered through teeth closed tightly in a frozen smile.

Mike was new to American culture, just off the plane so to speak, and he was genuinely puzzled. He asked, "Why not?"

"Just wait, you'll see."

I strode into the kitchen of his apartment and took a few really deep breaths before sweetly calling out, "Mike, may I see you in the kitchen for a moment please?"

His friends jabbed each other, smiling smugly. Mike came into the kitchen and asked me what was wrong. I grabbed him by his shirt front, backed him up against the refrigerator door, handed him the beer and said very quietly through clenched teeth, "If you ever snap your fingers at me again you'll find yourself a lot shorter than you are now. Got it?"

Having received a timely lesson in cultural diversity and too surprised to react, Mike took the beer out to his still nodding friends, a changed man.

From the fourth century to the Twentieth Century women were told their hair was their crowning glory, the essence of their beauty; but that essence was dangerously seductive, and therefore had to be hidden. The covering of women's hair became mandatory under the guise of religious law. Men considered their own temptation to be women's fault. Male self-control was not deemed to be male responsibility. Denied freedom, education and legal recourse, a woman could only accept what she was told by the men who had complete control over her life.

The log jam against a woman's right to her own being began to break up when Jesuit priests in North America saw how well matriarchal Indian societies worked. This new awareness of female intelligence and competency eventually changed a few male attitudes about the capabilities of women. Perhaps gender was not the issue after all. Perhaps the problem was lack of education and opportunity. It was a revolutionary, and very unpopular, theory.

At the same time, women in Europe, fed up with male control, were banding together to alter their personal and legal status. When Lincoln proclaimed American slaves to be free, suddenly a whole new stratum of repressed women seeking equality entered the fray. More about this in the next chapter.

And the Beat Goes On

If you think equating female baldness with shame is a thing of an ugly, archaic past, think again.

Remember Valerie, whose grandmother cut her hair just before graduation? That same Valerie had an educational business assignment in Iran in the early 1970's. She said she could just as easily have been on the French Riviera given the way women looked and dressed and cut their hair. Women were educators, judges, doctors—what-

BOLDLY BALD WOMEN

ever they could dream and would work to become.

Women's rights were effectively turned to dust after Ayatolla Khomeini took power in 1979 and dictated Sharia law to become the governing law of Iran. Women had to cover their bodies from head to toe, declaring them, once again, to be the temptresses and thereby declaring men, once again, not responsible for their own actions. If they wouldn't comply, Article 102 of Iran's constitution condemned them to seventy four strokes of the lash. Women once again could do nothing without permission from their husbands—including cutting their hair. But their husbands could divorce them without notice at anytime. So if a woman became bald, she was no longer valuable breeding stock. I divorce you, Baldy, and I, your now ex-husband, keep the kids.

Don't even get me started on what has happened to the women of Iran since the institution of Sharia law. This destruction goes way beyond the scope of a woman's right to cut her hair. The World Health Organization has established that Iran is the third top ranking country of death by suicide. In a western province of Iran, the deputy governor on women's affairs reported seventy percent of suicides in the province were women and ninety percent of those were between the ages of seventeen and thirty five years. The younger Iranian women who cherished their freedom have been completely devastated.

Do you think the United States, land of the free and home of the brave, is exempt from punishing women by shaving off their hair? Think again. On September 16, 2009 in Hillsborough County, Florida, a man was arrested for allegedly beating his young daughter with a belt and shaving her head as punishment for his belief that she had shoplifted jewelry from a Wal-Mart, and had taken a Game Boy from his room to play with it without his permission. School authorities reported possible child abuse when the girl came to school with her head shaved.

The father admitted to shaving the girl's head but denied the alleged beating. The man was accused of third-degree felony child abuse. Hillsborough County Sheriff's Office spokesman declared the charge was based primarily on the alleged beating and not on the shaving of the girl's head. The father was released on his own recognizance the following day. The questions asked by the blogger reprinting the story were, "What do you think? Is forcibly shaving a child's head just another type of punishment, or is it child abuse in the form of humiliation?" So . . . what do you think?

The effects of negative attitudes toward female baldness go beyond loss of hair to the very core of feminine identity. Increasing the connection between luxurious hair and feminine value has become the foundation of a global industry that grossed approximately $42.5 billion in 2010 and continues to increase revenue by leaps and bounds. The pressure is on to respect the hair. Is it any wonder the majority of bald women hide?

CHAPTER 4
Snake Oil

⤞⤝

*No amount of self-improvement
can make up for a lack of self-acceptance.*
—Anonymous

⤞⤝

Companies spend billions of dollars advertising their products. Why? It works. A world market for hair care products of $42.5 billion is a pretty big pie. Every hair care company out there wants a slice.

How do they get that slice? By convincing us we need their products in order to feel healthy, beautiful, sexy, worthy, secure, classy, and powerful—name your desire. All this, they insinuate, in addition to clean hair.

In 1915, when the bob haircut came into style, new products popped up like mushrooms in a compost heap. After centuries of elaborately braided, woven, and curled hair, straight hair was the *in* style. So many women were getting their hair cut, that men's barbers were inundated. The result? Women's beauty shops came into being.

At the same time, a whole new market developed for hair care of both genders of the African American community. They could signal their rising status through the visual language of hair. Straight hair became popularly known as *good hair*, and getting straight hair

BOLDLY BALD WOMEN

became the thing to do. The opportunistic advertisers were right there to reassure our black sisters and brothers they would surely feel healthy, beautiful, sexy, worthy, secure, classy, and powerful if they only used xyz hair care product.

What about women with no hair—whether from alopecia or poor nutrition? No worries, Mate. The products to cover a woman's bald head provided one more opportunity for companies to make money by appealing to the same emotions. Wigs of all types, materials, colors, and fashions became a huge business.

The advertising message was and is: let us help you keep your secret so you, too, you unfortunate woman, can *look* beautiful, healthy, sexy, worthy, secure, classy, powerful and feel safe from humiliation and rejection. Of course, the basic assumption was that bald women are *not* beautiful, healthy, sexy, worthy, secure, classy, powerful, and don't feel safe from humiliation and rejection. Now *there's* an assumption that needs revamping.

These days wigs and weaves and extensions are worn by celebrities who give the hair pieces even more appeal. The size of the market pie increases.

I imagine you are wondering why I think this isn't a win-win situation. Somebody sells something another person wants and everybody's happy. Oh, my dears, if only that were true. It's not the products themselves that I object to. It's the insidious undermining of a woman's personal value just as she is. A woman is good *if...* she is beautiful *if...* she is sexy *if...* on and on and on. Most of us not only buy the products, we buy into the hype as well.

All that hype is snake oil. Words and images (carefully couched to avoid law suits for false advertising) promise us emotional wholeness, inner peace, acceptance, and the good life if only we buy ... use ... do ... wear.

BOLDLY BALD WOMEN

While so many in the world live in the kind of poverty where a metal pot to cook in makes you wealthy, we live in a fantasy world where perfection of physical appearance is not simply a pastime, it is deemed a necessity. If it's flawed, cover it up. If it's broad, run it off or suck it out. If it's too long or too short or too big or too small, pay to have it cut and reshaped and re-sized.

Aging is not about increasing knowledge, wisdom, character, understanding and acceptance of self and others. It is about fighting the mortal enemies of lines and creases twenty-four hours a day. It is about hiding and constant vigilance. Difference is not to be explored and celebrated, it is to be camouflaged and minimized. Put this on. There, now only your hairdresser will know for sure.

Like the promise of cool water in a desert mirage, the promise of inner peace and contentment amid the constant covering up, primping, and making over is an illusion. The truth is we become more entrenched in the belief we are not good enough as we are. It is about believing our value comes not from our character and our actions, but rather from our ability to hide flaws.

I tried to swallow the snake oil promises when my hair fell out. I ended up choking. I bought the wig and wanted to believe it would fix the problem of my bald head. I began wearing makeup to fill in for missing eyebrows and minimize the alien look of missing eyelashes. I looked in the mirror and I saw a stranger, not myself. Not me without the wig and not me with the wig.

Writes Kristine—

For twelve years I searched for a miracle product that would cure hair loss. I spent a lot of money on products that claimed to cure hair loss and never did. I tried:

- Better nutrition

-Rogaine

BOLDLY BALD WOMEN

-*Minoxinale*
-*MSM*
-*Did head stands*
-*Aromatherapy*
-*Herbal teas*
-*Acupuncture*
-*Reflexology*

I would love to have all that money back for all those pills and potions and lotions. I could have taken a vacation to New Zealand with it. I would have been better off.

For myself—and many others—there had to be a better way. But what was it and how would I find it?

CHaPTeR 5
Wake Up and Smell the Hairspray

ॐ

*I don't know the key to success,
but the key to failure is to try to please everyone.*
—Bill Cosby

ॐ

People can be cruel. It's a fact of life. I wanted to sidestep this issue because the whole purpose of this book is to encourage you to let go of fear so you won't need to cling to wigs and scarves as though they can save you from discomfort. But, all the worry and anxiety, causing the hyper-vigilance necessary to keep those wigs and scarves in place and to protect your bald head from discovery, are holes in the bucket of your well-being. Worry and anxiety constantly drain your inner peace.

It is said our secrets keep us sick. I believe this. Still, if you look around and all you see are emotional machetes waiting to cut your head off, chances are you'll keep your secrets to save your neck. Therefore, not talking about the reality of cruelty won't help you be free. It is knowledge you need. Let's talk about the manifestations of emotional machetes, namely, cruelty.

There are different kinds of cruelty. They are worth looking at if you are a woman thinking about revealing your bald head to the world.

BOLDLY BALD WOMEN

The first type is cultural cruelty. This is prevalent where religious laws or mores forbid women from baring their heads for anyone but their husbands. In those places, women who have hair struggle. Women without hair are shunned, cast aside as being visibly punished by God for some transgression or other. They are considered evil and unhealthy. One woman wrote to me that in her country it was taboo to even speak of her baldness. She always kept her head covered no matter what the circumstance. Such cultural cruelty allows no respite from constant self-awareness. Being considered unacceptable by the very people who should love you no matter what is beyond sad.

The second type of cruelty comes from people who take a perverse delight in bullying others. As I believe in goodness, so I believe in evil. These are people who dwell so far from the light of love that anyone illuminated by love's light becomes repulsive and painful to them. These are men and women untouched by codes of morality and essentially without conscience. They are verbally and emotionally abusive. Whether or not we wear a wig is of little significance to them. We need to deal with them in any way necessary to keep ourselves safe and exert our human rights. This includes getting the law involved if and when it is necessary. This includes whistle blowing in a work setting. It must be made clear that there is zero tolerance for bullies.

The third kind of cruelty is reactive rather than deliberate. Most people who are cruel are so broken themselves that the concepts of acceptance, compassion, and nurturing are foreign, and painfully uncomfortable to them. They believe kindness is not to be trusted. They consider wholeness of spirit fraudulent, something to be countered with derision and disdain. They demand their own standards of perfection from everyone around them. Woe to those who don't or won't measure up.

BOLDLY BALD WOMEN

I had an uncle whose childhood left him negatively reactive to those he considered less than his definition of perfect. His reactionary behavior is explained by the fact that he was born with a cleft lip and palate. When he was a little boy, his father, who was a butcher by trade and afflicted with bipolar disorder, would chase after him with a cleaver whenever the father was drunk. He cursed and swore he could not have sired such an ugly monster. My uncle's father accused his wife of infidelity because of her baby's deformity. Eventually, my grandmother had enough, gathered up her children and divorced her cruel husband.

My uncle grew into a judgmental, controlling, perfectionist. His critical sarcasm toward the imperfections of others camouflaged his own unhealed pain and anger. If he could judge somebody else as less-than, he then became more-than. But, there was more to my uncle than his desire for perfection. He had successes and friendships in his life as well. He was a talented photographer who was able to provide for his family by his skill and creativity. For the people he truly cared about, he could lower his barriers. Those selected few found him to be pleasant company and a wonderful mentor. Still, his cruelty, a deadly accurate emotional machete, is the part of his character aimed at me when I was a young girl. I was overweight and plain and an unworthy subject for his photographic genius. His cruelty is all I remember him for. It is a sad legacy.

I don't think anybody gets through life without some emotional scars. It is part of the School of Life, part of the lessons we are on Earth to learn. We all have tender spots that hurt when poked. Our protective reactions can hurt those we care about just as their reactions to their own fear or pain can hurt us.

Reactive cruelty is malleable. Reactive cruelty can benefit from counseling and therapy. It can—if the person is willing to delve within—be examined and the cause identified. Emotional pain can be healed. Find and remove the thorn, treat it for infection, and pain fades. Though the scar remains, we are able to stop swiping at those who unintentionally bump into the site of the wound.

Remember jO, the second generation holocaust survivor whose extended family were decimated in the death camps of Germany during World War II? The first time jO's father saw her after she shaved her head, he was devastated. His unsupportive negativity was excruciating to jO as she tried to deal with her own pain. She had looked to her father for understanding and acceptance.

Here was a man for whom bald heads, especially on women, were associated with the basest kind of degradation, dehumanization and decimation. The heads of all prisoners were shaved in the death camps for protection against lice and as a means of humiliation. After World War II, the heads of women accused of collaborating with the Germans were shaved to publicly humiliate and shame them. The women were ridiculed, spat upon and beaten and often tarred and feathered if they had worked for or prostituted themselves to the German soldiers—even if they did so to prevent being shot, or to keep their children from starving. Bald was definitely not beautiful for jO's father. Not beautiful. Not acceptable. But eventually his love for his daughter, and his understanding of her need to be free from the tyranny of her own secret shame, enabled him to temper his deeply ingrained revulsion and come to a place of acceptance.

That's an extreme case to be sure. Still, there are many people out there who have great personal pain behind their negative reactions to female baldness. Perhaps their pain is a loved one lost to cancer. Perhaps, like jO's father, they have a fear of reliving past terrors. That doesn't mean we denigrate ourselves and cover our heads to protect those around us from their personal pain. It means once we realize we're protecting them from their own issues, we stop hurting ourselves to rescue others from their own discomfort. We can't live happily in our own lives when we deny our own reality. Take for example, my sister, who I love, more than life itself.

My Sister's Hats

My sister was eleven years old when I was born. When I was five, our mother went back to work as a registered nurse in a local hospital. My sister was the built-in babysitter. I was the built-in chaperone for many of her dates. Whether I tagged along when she went to the beach, or tip-toed over squeaky kitchen floor boards to spy as she and her beau said a prolonged good night at the back door landing, I was a royal pain in her neck. My sister was very frustrated by having to play surrogate mother while our mom was at work. Although I'll deny it completely if you tell her, I was often a belligerent brat. It is quite understandable that I was twenty-six before she finally made up her mind in favor of letting me live out the sum of my God-given years.

Our father died when I was sixteen, and our mother died when I was thirty-five and living abroad in Greece with my husband. Some years after our only brother died, and I had survived a potentially fatal bout with ovarian cancer, I asked my sister if she was glad she'd chosen not to strangle me on any one those numerous occasions she believed me deserving of immediate death.

"Most days I am," she said. "Why?"

"It turns out I'm the only member of our nuclear family you've got left."

She visibly startled. "I hadn't thought of it that way. You're right," she said softly.

"What? I'm WHAT? I'm right? Right?"

I bolted to the wall calendar and wrote on the day's date in per-

49

manent Sharpie marker: "PAM WAS RIGHT!" As I returned to our Canadian Canasta game, she swatted me playfully in sisterly pique and we continued together to soundly trounce our husbands at cards.

What does that story have to do with living boldly bald? More than anybody in my life, my sister suffered the emotional trauma of my hair loss. She wouldn't look at me. She would turn away or cover her eyes with her hand whenever I took off the wig.

"Cover your head!" she'd insist, and I would, understanding, but feeling frustrated and hurt. When it became clear that wigs simply were not for me either physically or emotionally, she frowned, pursed her lips and said: "Well, then start wearing hats."

"Sister-mine," I retorted, "if you want me to wear hats, you'd better get busy and make them."

Darned if she didn't find several crocheted hat patterns and do just that! Each new hat was an experiment in style and color and materials. Each one was better than the one before. Each one got jazzed up with broaches and flowers and buttons and doo-dahs. They are fun and stylish and sassy. We've found I'm happiest with a fedora that has wire in the rim so I can shape it to my whim of the day. A fedora suits my last-of-the-red-hot-mama's-despite-being-old-and-fat swagger.

The day my sister came to accept me as bald was the day I took off my hat to mop pooling sweat. She saw how sopping wet the paper towel became.

"I can't do this anymore," I said in distress. "I can't be this uncomfortable to protect you from your distaste."

She looked stunned. Turns out, it wasn't distaste—it was both fear and her sense of propriety. If my sister didn't see the baldness, she wouldn't have to see the stark difference in how I looked. She wouldn't have to cope with something being wrong or worry that she might lose me.

BOLDLY BALD WOMEN

Where I have always been outgoing and in-your-face-Snoopy-happy-dance effervescent, my sister has always been a reserved and private person. When we went places together and my head was covered, she didn't have to cope with as many stares or potential looks or questions that might hurt me, and she could relax and enjoy our outing. She is my big sister. She was protecting me.

Somewhere along the line we both realized that I can't live my life from the perspective of my sister's comfort—or anyone else's. She reluctantly left her comfort zone behind and looked openly at my bald head. She hugged me and touched the baby bottom softness of my scalp without flinching. My sister said she made the decision to be okay with my baldness. She said it, but I knew it was her love for me speaking. I knew she really meant it the day she told me if I wanted any more hats I'd have to learn how to make them myself. I cherish the hats my sister made me. I wear them often in the cold Michigan winters for warmth, and style, and the soul-surrounding comfort of her heartfelt caring.

Hat's on—and off—to you, sister-mine! I love you too, more than I have words to say and more than you have ears to hear. I love you all the way to the moon and back a bazillion times over. Now I've done it. She's blushing and blustering. Good thing she's already decided to let me live.

There is one more type of cruelty I want to mention before we move on. That is the unintentional cruelty of ignorance and thoughtless curiosity. This is my favorite kind of cruelty. This is where my bald head truly shines. These are the stares of little children in the supermarket as they point and whisper to their parents to look at the bald lady. This is the furtive glances of those parents and the inevitable "Shhh." I enjoy these moments, because I know each one is another opportunity to use curiosity to combat ignorance.

51

BOLDLY BALD WOMEN

Casually, I speed up until I am alongside the child and say, "I noticed you are looking at my head. I bet you saw I don't have any hair, right?"

There is an awestruck nod and a glance at mom or dad, who usually look uncomfortably embarrassed and toss an apology at me for their child's lack of manners.

"Do you know why I don't have any hair?" A wide-eyed side to side shake of the head follows. I go into my children's version of Alopecia 101, and in this way I educate both child and parents while making fast friends with the children. They wave and sometimes blow kisses every time our carts pass in the aisles during the rest of the shopping trip.

Yes, I know, the looks and the murmurs can be annoying when it's the thirty-seventh time that week. I know there are occasions when we just don't have the wear-with-all or the time to educate the world about alopecia. But for me, it has become a life calling. I owe my avocation to a beautiful, five-year-old girl sitting in the child seat of her mother's shopping cart with her curly blond hair pulled back into an unruly pony tail. She looked at me with such sad brown eyes that I simply had to speak with her. I went into my spiel about noticing her noticing my head and asked her if she knew why I didn't have any hair.

Her eyes filled with tears. She nodded slowly and whispered, "Yes. You are going to die."

Her answer stunned me. The little girl's mother quickly intervened. She shared that her daughter's best friend had recently died of cancer after going through chemotherapy and losing all her hair. The mother's anxious eyes pleaded with me not to take offense.

"Oh, honey," I soothed, "I'm so sorry about your friend. You must have loved her very much and miss her now."

BOLDLY BALD WOMEN

She nodded, tears spilling down pale cheeks. "When you have a bald head you die," she said in sorrowful certainty.

"Oh, sweetheart, I know it must seem that way, but I'm not dying. I just have a body that is a little confused. It thinks my hairs are bad guys and kicks them out of my body and won't let them grow back again."

"Why?"

"Nobody really knows yet, but the doctors are working to find out. I want you to remember that not everybody with a bald head has cancer. And, even though some of the bald people do have cancer, the medicine they take to help them get well is very strong and sometimes makes their hair fall out. But not everyone with a bald head will die. I had cancer a long time ago, and I didn't die. People who have cancer work hard to get better. And the doctors work hard to help them get better too. Many of the people who have cancer will get better and their hair will grow back after awhile. My hair probably won't ever grow back, but I'm not sick and I'm not sad about having no hair. It's actually kind of cool because..."

Then I went into the part about no shampoo stinging my eyes, no tangles to comb through, no having to sit still while mommy braids my hair, no trying to wipe hair out of my eyes when I'm all sweaty from playing hard—all the things kids hate about hair when they aren't busy looking at themselves in the mirror pretending to be princesses and princes or Wonder Women and rappers, or whatever they pretend these days. At the end of our talk she dried her eyes and was smiling. I hadn't healed the hurt of her lost friend, but I had given her hope and made her laugh.

There is a saying: Do what you can where you are with what you have.

My baldness is what I have that makes me different from other women. I didn't ask for it, but I choose to use that difference as a

BOLDLY BALD WOMEN

lighthouse beacon, revealing a path to understanding and acceptance. I choose to use it as a source of hope. I choose to use it to
prove that nights of loss and grief have no power to hide the way to
self-acceptance and joy. I choose to use it to show that when we use
our courage and strength, we can move out of isolation and misery. I
choose to use my difference to guide bald women towards self-love,
and towards acceptance of the foibles of others, without accepting
their judgments or their preferences as the truth.

Dear hearts, what will you choose to do with your baldness?

CHAPTER 6
The Sixty-Four Thousand Dollar Question

೨∘ல

The privilege of a lifetime is being who you are.
—Joseph Campbell

೨∘ல

During the 1960's, there was a television game show where the host asked a series of increasingly difficult questions. The prize money doubled with each correctly answered question until the contestants reached the final level with the hardest question: the sixty four thousand dollar question. The phrase became slang for a particularly difficult question or problem.

So here's the sixty four thousand dollar question for bald women:

Why, given cruelty towards and discrimination against women daring to go bald in public, would any woman in her right mind expose herself to the emotional discomfort and social intolerance of female baldness?

Some might answer: no woman in her right mind would make that decision. However, *au contraire, mon amie*, there are some excellent reasons why a woman of sound mind would choose to be boldly bald.

BOLDLY BALD WOMEN

The first reason is physical comfort. Wigs are hot and itchy. Wearing a wig makes most women who wear them unavoidably self-conscious. Contrast that with a man who, if he's going bald, simply shaves his head to become both physically and socially cool with the same razor stroke. Look around at all the bald men in the movies and magazines, on the streets, and in your extended family. Nobody gives it a second thought. So why shouldn't balding women have the same option of achieving that physical comfort? Exactly, there is no reason they shouldn't.

The second reason is freedom of choice. Not all women will choose to be boldly bald. I'm not suggesting they must or even should. Whether for personal preference or for religious reasons, those who choose to cover their heads certainly have every right to do so—just as do men when they choose to wear hair pieces. It's not about the choice one makes. It's about the right to choose without fear of derision or discrimination.

That right doesn't come cheap. Pioneering women pay the price every day. They brave the gauntlet of emotional rejection, ridicule, prejudice, lost opportunities for promotion at best or lost relationships and employment at worst, taunting, physical bullying, mistaken gender identity, confusion with cancer survivors, misidentification with the often violent youth subculture of white-supremacist skin heads, religious faction disapproval and historical bias.

Remember the women who had no right to even cut their own hair? Remember the suffragettes—women joining women (and many savvy and secure men) to fight for voting rights? And the women's equal rights and the gay rights movements in the Seventies that walked both in step with, and on the heels of, the civil rights movement? There is always a price to pay when fighting for change.

The difference between those movements and today's boldly

BOLDLY BaLD Women

bald women's movement is visibility and proximity. Yes, there are over five million people with alopecia in the United States alone. About fifty percent of them are women. But most of those two-and-a-half million women are invisible via deliberate hiding. Many of those women never reveal their baldness. Standing alone is a lot more intimidating and leaves women more vulnerable than facing social hostility with a host of like-minded people. There is power in numbers.

The overwhelming sense of being alone is the number one feeling women have related to me about dealing with hair loss. That's a long way from the "we're-in-this-together" camaraderie of those other movements. Courageous women around the world are daring to step across the line from acceptable hiding, which, by the way, does not equate to pain-free existence, to unacceptable shining. One here, one there—women who once believed themselves to be alone now feel freer to challenge the status quo in their personal relationships, work environments, schools, churches, on city streets and in every social setting.

Of course, in today's world the Internet affects the potential success of this movement. Women are finding Alopecia World and the National Alopecia Areata Foundation through the Internet. These organizations bring together women with alopecia from all around the world. Suddenly, they're not alone anymore. Suddenly, there are whole communities of people of both genders who understand—people who live with hair loss every day. There are many who have insight to offer. They have solutions to problems and tips on increasing community understanding and social acceptance. These are people who get the importance of sharing stories.

Women, like the ones who graciously participated in the creation of this book, know we must have stories to share in order to teach, and to support our sisters in the throes of dealing with hair loss

BOLDLY BALD WOMEN

trauma. Such women have learned to love themselves and their bald-ness—and yes, even come prefer it Such women understand there can be no life-changing, uplifting stories of hope for our sisters without the courage to live life openly as a boldly bald woman. They hold their heads high. They smile with confidence. They exhibit gracious understanding for traumatic first reactions of family, friends, employers, employees, and the general public. Didn't we all experience traumatic first reactions to ourselves when we lost our hair? Women with a straightforward spirit are ready to invite questions. They are also uniquely prepared with short, easy-to-understand answers when others ask the inevitable questions.

There are amazing women in the world who understand that our baldness gives us an opportunity to step out of our comfort zones to become ambassadors for baldness. We are the changers of perception who will benefit not only Alopecians, but also all women who face baldness for whatever reason in whatever season of their lives. These are women who understand that we live in exciting times. They understand how incredibly cool it is that we take part in an historical change every bit as significant as the suffragettes, civil rights, and gay rights movements.

If you think I'm exaggerating, imagine how different your city would look if there were as many openly bald women as there are men. And, imagine the positive change on the self-esteem of those women and how that change would impact their personal and professional relationships. Imagine the impact freedom from ridicule and persecution would have on each succeeding generation. Those future girls and boys who today must deal with the ridicule of baldness as vulnerable children, would not experience the intolerance that children do today.

If you think the courage of the few to stand up to the many as advocates for open female baldness is not important, if you think this

58

battle is a tempest in a teapot, then go back again to the statistics of how many millions of women have alopecia worldwide. Add to those numbers the women who, though the advances of technology in our fight against cancer, deal with baldness while they are fighting for their very lives. Do you think they also need the negativity directed toward bald women? And what about the young children who deal with hair loss just as their sense of self-value is developing? What if no hair was just another style—like pony tails or corn rows or weaves or pixie cuts? Who will make that perception become the accepted reality, if we don't?

There is a third reason for women to risk living openly with baldness. Sometimes unexpectedly wonderful things happen. Here are the stories of women who decided to make a bold change and some of the things that happened as a result. They come from women of all ages, religions and cultures from all over the world. It is a global community.

❖ *There was a lot of consideration that went into my decision to ditch the wig. When I had moved to Guelph, Ontario we finally got the Internet and I discovered alopecia groups on yahoo and msn. I had never really met anyone else with alopecia (except a high school friend's mom who avoided talking about it) and it was inspiring to see pictures of all these happy, bald alopecians who led normal lives. Socially this was difficult for my mate as he never had to deal with rude stares and comments; however it slowly became easier for both of us.*

I received much praise from my online communities and am grateful they were there for me to aid my growth. Meeting other Alopecians is something I've been doing more lately since I decided I have grown and become strong enough to lead a support group.

BOLDLY BALD WOMEN

I was also lucky enough to have lunch with a group of ladies in Toronto and experienced seeing bald women like me for the first time. It did take a few years to achieve my current comfort level. I began slowly going out bald in my backyard where only a few neighbors might see, then to the mall where I had to deal with my new image when I got questioned or stared at.

Since the beginning of a new Web site called Alopecia World, I have enjoyed a few great opportunities and continue to be an inspiration to Alopecians all over the world. I have written for another book and a Dutch magazine about alopecia. My support group has just celebrated its one year anniversary and the Children's Alopecia Project (CAP) asked me to be guest speaker at their conference. I did a music workshop with the kids, teaching them how to express themselves when no one around them "gets it." The thing that inspired me the most now is hearing about the kids with alopecia sharing their condition with not just their class but their entire school. This really seems to help them and is something I wish I could have done had it been acceptable at the time. There are so many young people with alopecia who have amazing attitudes! Second to that, I am always happy to see another bald lady come to terms with her condition and go "AU-natural" as someone once put it.

We still have a long way to go before people stop assuming we're chemotherapy patients or understand that bald can be attractive too and that is why I will always do everything possible to put us on the fast track to awareness and acceptance.

—Carol J.

❖ *To be free, comfortable, confident, happy and striving in self acceptance. Be who you are. Never allow anyone to step into your shoes with their opinions of how your life should pan out.*

BOLDLY BALD WOMEN

—jO

❖ *Nothing prompted me. It's a process. I received a great amount of encouragement from family, co-workers and friends. The support from other Alopecians on AlopeciaWorld.com has been instrumental to my self-acceptance and courage to go out bald in public . . . I'm not embarrassed when I'm bald in public, but there are times when I am painfully self-conscious. Sometimes I feel like I'm floating; I found out that was a symptom of anxiety.*

—Galena

❖ *For Catholics, Lent is the beginning of when you give up something, you make a sacrifice. I realized that I was holding onto the fear of being rejected and being vulnerable because I was bald and hid behind my wigs. I realized that I needed to give up that fear.*

—Caitlin

❖ *The level of discomfort, especially in the summer. And photos of women who do not wear head coverings and are so beautiful.*

—April

❖ *My spiritual teacher encouraged me to begin my path without my wig. She encouraged baby steps. Since I hardly ever went out, I could start with a kerchief. One afternoon, I thought I'd take a walk around my neighborhood bare headed and was shocked at how rude people truly are. I barely walked a kilometer, and three people had made rude comments at me: "Nice hair!" "Did you use a lawnmower to shave that?" "Do you really think that hair your haircut makes you look good?"*

BOLDLY BALD WOMEN

I was heartbroken, but my very wise child said to me: "Don't let them stop your progress, Mom. Hang in there, they're just jerks and you're gonna always have a few jerks." My daughter buzzed all her hair off in support of me, and kept saying, it's just hair mom. No wonder she is often my inspiration!

After that, I would dress pretty and go for a walk at our lake which has a boardwalk. I tried to feel like a million dollars, and was actually treated well, as people did stare, but I tried to tell myself it was because I looked good rather than bald.

—Willow

❖ *When I first lost my hair, I refused to wear a wig because I felt that would admit defeat to the disease. But after a year, when my hair didn't grow back, I began to wear them. However, they were hot and itchy, especially in the summertime.*

I was searching on the internet one night to see if there were any new developments in treatments for alopecia, and came across the website AlopeciaWorld.com. Through this networking site I found so many other people with my condition. I found out I wasn't alone in this world. Some of the friends I made there go out bald headed, and I gained a lot of courage from those ladies.

It took eight full years to come to full acceptance of alopecia. It started after the birth of my youngest daughter. You see, it was one of those two AM feedings. As she was dozing in my arms, I thought about how everything happens for a reason. I remembered someone once telling me that I am God's creation, and, as such, I am beautiful. I realized that I really hated my bald appearance, and that is a terrible way to feel about myself.

That night, I bowed my head and prayed for God to forgive me for being so embarrassed by my appearance. I truly believe ev-

erything happens for a reason. From that moment on, it was a slow inward process of accepting myself as I am. I remember going outside without my head covered for the first time. I actually had to consciously give myself permission to do so. Now, I love being unique and I celebrate the person I am created to be!

On my eighth anniversary of hairlessness I put my wigs aside and decided that God made me bald for a reason—I don't have any idea what that reason could be, but I finally chose not to hide my bald head anymore. And boy, wig-free is a comfortable way to be!

Before alopecia, I saw myself as quiet. I was shy and timid and very nervous about talking to people. A true introvert, who didn't like to go out in public. Since accepting my alopecia and becoming a Boldly Bald Woman, I have become much more outgoing! Now, I see myself as someone who can handle just about anything that comes my way. I think that others see me as strong—epecially once they see that I am happy with myself.

I am happy being bald. I celebrate my uniqueness. So, even if they found a cure for alopecia now, I wouldn't take it. I like me the way I am. I want you to know that in spite of starting off with alopecia sad, scared, and embarrassed to be bald, I write to you today happy and strong, and proud to be the person I am. Alopecia universalis has not been the end, but a brand new beginning for me. And joy really DOES return in the morning. Life is good—hair or no hair.

—Sandy K.

❖ *Wigs are really uncomfortable, hot and itchy. And, I like being bald. I got involved with other women who have this. I do find some women to be very gorgeous bald. That's what gorgeous earrings are for and lots of eye makeup. Men have struggled to have that comfort level for themselves, and I do the bald look so it becomes an option for me and other gals.*

—Carol S.

❖ *I had enough of the restrictions that came with wig wearing. I have an active lifestyle. I felt ready to ditch my comfort blanket and grow up as an Alopecian. I am what I am. My partner was instrumental in giving me the courage to be just me and my daughter was also full of encouragement. She gave her English class a presentation on alopecia and I felt incredibly proud.*

—Sharan

❖ *The final blow came when wig number four ripped in half. I went on a week's girls' holiday to Cyprus, where I plucked up the courage to go without anything on my head. I decided that now was the time to go bald and especially just a few days away from International Alopecia Day. My first day back at work after my holiday was very nerve racking, and even though most people knew I had alopecia, revealing my bald head had been something very personal to me over the last seven years. Once I had done it, I felt a huge sense of empowerment. Colleagues, friends and family have all been fantastic and given me the confidence to go for it.*

—Gwennan

❖ *When my alopecia began to progress rapidly I became very depressed, cried a lot and constantly checked my head for expansion of the bald areas. I began to move forward only when I shaved my head. Shaving gave me control and I stopped worrying about losing my hair once it was all gone. I decided not to wear a wig*

*simply because of the physical discomfort. I had too many experi-
ences of having sweat run down my head under the wig and excess
body heat. On more than one occasion I ended up tearing the wig
off in anger and crying.*

*I feel strongly that not wearing a head covering and appear-
ing in public bald is a feminist issue. Men with hair loss shave
their heads and we see them everywhere. Bald men appear in
fashion ads and in movies. People don't assume that bald men
have cancer, and no one stares at a man because he's bald. Women
should have the same choice to go bald that men do, and not be
forced to endure hot and uncomfortable head coverings.*

—Mary

❖ *When Olivia lost all of her hair the second time I had a custom wig made for her. We planned a 'Hair Party' at the company
that supplied the hair system. I invited all of our friends and family to see Olivia's 'reveal'. She looked amazing; however Olivia
did not like wearing her hair. At age 8, she was too young to deal
with the glue that was used to attach the hair to her head. After
3 months of wearing it, she woke up one morning and announced
that she was going to school without her hair. I was shocked and
spoke to her teacher, the school nurse, the school counselor and the
after school YMCA counselors. Everyone was in agreement; we
had to allow Olivia to do this her way. She went to school that day
bald and has been publicly bald since then.*

—Sandy R.

❖ *It was very hard in my early years living with alopecia areata. I was in denial and avoided mirrors and just hoped no one
would notice it enough to point it out to me. I soon noticed when*

people were talking to me they were always looking at the ever-so-balding part straight down the left side of my head. And my fiancé (now husband) brought it up in conversation one day. He could see it clearly because he is taller than I am. All this time I was just hoping it wouldn't get noticed.

I just got tired of obsessing about it. My fiancé and I were living and working in Yellowstone National Park—the most beautiful place on earth and all I can think of is my hair loss. I told myself this had to stop. I wanted to shave it off. Out of sight, out of mind. My release. Set me free! And it worked. It felt so good. No hair. No need for so called miracle products. Gone. Now I can be here in the present and enjoy my life! I am perfectly healthy – good mind – good heart – okay body (work in progress). It's just hair.

Turned out I felt kind of sexy. My fiancé was totally turned on by it. I'm happy. He's happy. Life is good. The list of reasons I decided not to wear a wig?

1. *They itch.*
2. *I can spot a wig a mile and a half away.*
3. *Can't afford the expensive ones.*
4. *Doesn't fit my lifestyle.*
5. *If I'm bike riding and the wind decides to blow really hard and blows the wig off my head I'm not the type to turn around and go after it.*
6. *Same goes for hiking.*
7. *I enjoy driving fast and feeling the wind on my face. Can't do this while wearing a wig.*
8. *Requires too much maintenance and hair products – again!*
9. *I'm happier without one*

BOLDLY BALD WOMEN

10.   Plan on starting a revolution of bald men and women and cats and dogs and all other hairless animals. Viva la bald! It's already started. This book proves it.

—Kristine

CHAPTER 7
Alopecia World

᷿᷍

Do not follow where the path may lead.
Go, instead, where there is no path and leave a trail.
—Ralph Waldo Emerson

᷿᷍

When I first lost my hair, I was Alice in Not-So-Wonderland chasing after the white rabbit of there-IS-a-better-way-than-hiding. I fell through a cyber-net hole into the wonderland called Alopecia World and landed with a click. Everywhere I turned, men, women, and children were coping with hair loss—in all stages of all types of alopecia, as well as people who had lost hair from chemotherapy, hormonal problems, drug reactions and trichotillomania (uncontrollable hair pulling). Here anxious, hurting newcomers were welcomed with acceptance, empathy, and information. Here they could access the wisdom of those who had coped with hair loss for many years.

I learned my shiny, bald head is in the company of a myriad of delightful people worldwide. While some women are only interested in how to best hide their baldness, many others believe that as there is room for bald men, there is also room for bald women and children of all ages and backgrounds. Their stories are as diverse as the women themselves—stories that weave together into an elegant tapestry depicting courage, humor and strength in the face of adversity.

BOLDLY BALD WOMEN

Alopecia World

Cheryl Carvery-Jones launched Alopecia World early in 2007 with her truly wonderful husband, RJ. Cheryl's courage in facing her own baldness and her determination to use her difference to help other women cope with baldness became the springboard to an ever expanding global community of women, children and men.

Alopecia World provides a forum for discussions in such categories as:

Acceptance and coping
Bald is beautiful
Children with alopecia
Employment issues, workplace challenges
Events, special announcements
Gender issues
In the news, media, publications
Inspirational, motivational
Just for fun
Love and relationships
Member spotlight
Promoting alopecia awareness
Society, culture, politics
Support groups
Symptoms, treatment options, research
Wigs, eyebrows, hair pieces, fashion

In Alopecia World there are sub-groups for children, teens, women, men, the different types of alopecia, various regions and states in the US, and many countries around the world. There are unrestricted sites within Alopecia World that can be accessed by those who don't have alopecia, but are looking to support someone who does, or to receive support themselves as they learn how to cope with changes in the person they care about. Alopecia World serves as a hub for people facing similar issues. One woman in England was feeling alone and discouraged. She wondered if there was another bald woman in or near her city. There was. They found each other on Alopecia World, chose to meet for lunch, and became close, mutually supportive friends.

Just who is this woman whose vision enabled a global community? How did she arrive at a place where she could cope openly with baldness? Cheryl tells her story.

Awakening to My Dream
Alopecia Totalis Meets Total Acceptance

I stood there gripping the doorknob, terribly afraid of walking out the door, and just as afraid of not doing so. I knew that as soon as I closed the door behind me, my life would never be the same. For the first time in a very long time, I was going to walk out the door being fully me, and I had no doubt that I would come back exhilarated and determined or exasperated and defeated.

I also knew that my friends and others were going to react, so I wondered how much negative feedback I might be able to handle. If they didn't like the new me, would I simply return home, place a wig back on my head, and go back to hiding? Needless to say, these thoughts were the scariest.

Undeterred, I made the courageous decision to walk out the door and reveal my bald head to my friends and even strangers. I couldn't have been more surprised by my friends' acceptance and encouragement as well as my own feelings that night.

For the first time in years, I was not afraid of crowds. I didn't worry that someone's wristwatch or necklace would be caught in my wig and carry it away, or that when someone hugged me, they might accidentally pull on my wig and expose my secret. The entire set of worries I usually carried were no longer there, and I was truly able to enjoy myself. Most importantly, I finally felt free and like me again.

Obviously, I came home pleased that I had ventured out without a wig. Nonetheless, it took me a while longer to settle on my new look. Therefore, over the next few years, I continued experimenting with wigs, hats and scarves. I also sported the au naturel look more and more until I eventually concluded that I prefer not covering my head at all.

Initially, I thought that I could pull off the bald look only while wearing jeans and a tank top. However, after I realized that the concept of femininity is a social construction that I can refashion to the satisfaction of my own sanity, strength and self-esteem, I found it very gratifying to create a womanly look with what some think is a man's hairdo. I came to realize that a woman could be bald, bold, and beautiful in a business suit, dress, or a pair of jeans. I truly began to appreciate what I saw in my mirror.

Reactions to my choice are not always positive. Sometimes a person has the audacity to suggest that I let whatever hair I have grow back and cover the remaining spots, or that I would look good (normal) in a nice wig. I've also been mistaken for a man, and I can tell the opinion of some people by the way they shamefully look away when I make eye contact with them. Regardless, I no longer feel like I'm hiding and I have no desire to go back to that place.

BOLDLY BALD WOMEN

My bald head may still attract some negative attention, but what's infinitely more important to me is that it attracts positive attention, too. It seems to make me approachable to people with questions and concerns about female baldness, or who are living with the same or a similar type of alopecia. Indeed, I'm often reminded that my freedom and confidence have also encouraged many women, especially female alopecians and cancer patients, to consider the bald and beautiful look as an alternative to wearing wigs and other head covers.

On the other hand, I really struggled with the whole idea of dating. When I was an independent, single woman, I was completely comfortable with my choice not to wear a wig. This was my decision and I couldn't have been happier with it. I didn't want any man to have any say regarding my alopecian style because I feared that doing so would jeopardize my freedom.

I maintained this wall of protection by keeping men at a distance. However, while not having to bother with their opinions of my alopecia made my life somewhat easier, it also made my life lonely. Years passed before I realized that my approach to coping with alopecia was more about avoidance and resignation than complete self-acceptance and the realization that I could still live life to the fullest while thoroughly enjoying a relationship with a man who truly appreciates the way I look as well as the way I am.

This new and liberating perspective on dating was confirmed when I met my husband, RJ, who helped me launch Alopecia World.com. Having opened myself to loving and being loved by him, I discovered that I could preserve my freedom even in the context of the most intimate of human relationships. The key in this regard has not only been his sensitivity to my feelings, but also my conscious effort to avoid being overly sensitive to his thoughts and feelings about my alopecia. To truly know that I'm not sleeping with the enemy is to truly understand that there's no need for me to spend every waking moment on the defensive.

When I was diagnosed with alopecia, everything I did was to avoid being stared at or thought of as different—from the Rogaine treatments I thought would re-grow my hair, to the wigs and lies I used in an effort to make sure no one learned my secret.

Today, I no longer cover my head. In fact, I hate doing so. I now accentuate my alopecia like I would any other part of my body that makes me uniquely me. Being "alopecic and adorable," as my husband says, has given me many opportunities to let my light shine. This head tells a story and needs to be displayed, not hidden.

Cheryl and RJ used their experience coping with baldness and technical savvy to create a forum in which anyone with hair loss can share their own struggles and insights, ask questions and get practical input—a haven of total acceptance, understanding and sometimes raucous humor. Alopecia World has become a very large, very eclectic, rapidly growing global village.

Most of the stories in this book have come from women I met through Alopecia World. Some are still trying to accept their own baldness. Others have gone beyond personal acceptance to working for international awareness and change. Their stories are crucial to other women facing baldness. Their stories are equally valuable to everyone who knows, is a friend to, lives with, loves, works with, or goes to school with a bald woman or girl.

Here is just one of the many positive connections which Alopecia World has enabled.

It was truly a glorious day for me! I admit I was a bit nervous about going bald in public in the beginning. My knees were all wobbly and I couldn't stop shaking, but after that, I got over it and I even walked around the high street alone for a good hour. I felt more confident than I ever was before. I thought people would be judgmental, but, in fact, it was the exact opposite. I got a lot of smiles and people were much, much nicer to me than I expected. A guy actually said hello to me and told me I was gorgeous! It was such a breakthrough. I have waited for what seems like forever for this moment to come. I am glad I met someone who is so courageous and oozes confidence. Thank you, Margaret. You made me feel so beautiful and helped me find the courage to face the world as I am. For that I am very, very grateful. And for those of you who are still unsure about going out in public bald, well these things take time, and I am sure that , like me, you will find the courage to say, 'Sod it! People should accept me for who I am and not by the way I look!' Good luck to all of you and I hope to see you in the near future.

—Salmeszan

Wow! I have at long last met up with an Alopecian—just like me. It was awesome! I chatted for hours to Salmeszan (Sal), who was also living near my home town and who—just like me—thought no one else was just like her. This was the first time in my entire life I met someone as brave as Sal in the flesh. I was so proud of Sal. For the first time ever, she took off her scarf and walked down the high street of Exeter with me. She said it was most uplifting, and I was overjoyed to have been there to support her. I wish I had been that brave when I was twenty-eight. It took me until I was forty! So come on everyone, be brave and show the world who we really are!

——Margaret

BOLDLY BALD WOMEN

Interactions like this are happening worldwide as a result of the efforts of Cheryl and RJ and are typical of the gift of community they provide for Alopecians.

Ignorant and non-supportive environments are locks that would prevent bald women from gaining admittance to the kind of acceptance experienced by bald men in our society. Self-acceptance and courage are the keys. More and more women are finding their keys and using them to gain personal freedom and change our society's perception of female baldness from the bizarre to the commonplace.

Have you found your key, yet? If you have, you are in for interesting insights into what others are doing with the self-acceptance and courage they have gained. If you haven't found your key, you are in the right place.

CHAPTER 8
The Most Excellent NAAF

సౌ✍

Excellence is the result of caring more than others think wise,
risking more than other's think safe,
dreaming more than others think practical,
and expecting more than others think possible.
—Anonymous

సౌ✍

Just as there is more than one way to get where you are going, there is more than one organization shining a light on the acceptability of baldness. Established in 1981, the National Alopecia Areata Foundation, NAAF, is an award-winning foundation that supports research for the cure or acceptable treatment of alopecia areata, supports those who have it, and educates the public about alopecia.

My first encounter with NAAF was the twenty-fifth annual conference held at the Hyatt Regency Hotel in Indianapolis, Indiana, in June of 2010. I was both a participant and a co-facilitator for the session called Free to be Bare. It was an amazing, tremendously empowering opportunity to meet and hug the people I had befriended around the country via the Internet. It was also a great opportunity to meet new friends.

To give you perspective into the impact of a NAAF conference, I'll tell you about a game my husband and I play when we go out to dinner. We live in Grand Rapids, the largest city in Western Michigan, with an estimated 2012 population of 190,000 (probably a few more since I wrote this sentence). Based on the formula of 1.2 percent of people actually presenting symptoms of alopecia at any one time, and just a bit over half being female, there are approximately 1,145 females presenting with some symptoms of alopecia in my city. Of course, not everyone will have alopecia universalis like I do, but there are many out there who are completely bald.

Our game begins on those rare occasions when we eat dinner at an especially nice restaurant with ambiance. The glow of gentle lighting falls softly on the heads of dining patrons to soothe away the day's stress and facilitate a relaxed, enjoyable evening meal. If one is fortunate, there might be enough light to actually see what is on the plate.

One thing that must be said for bald heads is they are very efficient light reflectors. While waiting for salads or soup, Mike and I look around and count the number of bald head reflections. Then, we determine the gender of the owner of the bald head. To date, wherever, whenever, mine has been the only female bald head.

How do I feel about that? Although it is a bit lonely, I feel privileged to be a pioneer. I imagine that must have been how the early suffragettes felt. I have been known to pick out a likely fellow on my way to the restroom, tap him on the shoulder, smile my biggest, happiest smile, and say, "Nice haircut." The looks I get when the people at his table look up are priceless.

The best response so far has been from a quick witted fellow who, without missing a beat, quipped, "Wow! Yours is good looking too. It's a lot closer than mine. Who's your barber?" We both laughed while the people around table blinked owlishly in stunned, hairy, silence. That's what I call acceptance with grace! It seems to be so much easier for bald men to find the humor in self-acceptance of bald women than for those men and women who haven't dealt with hair loss themselves. My hunch is, bald men have experienced a similar kaleidoscope of feelings and have thrown out the definition that bald means sick or unattractive.

The people at NAAF conferences take the 'what if' of bald women and children going without head coverings just as casually as most bald men do. As a result, being bald is a safe and happy reality for everyone who chooses it at the conference.

Everyone deals with alopecia in their own way and their own time frame. Some women are uncomfortable ever showing their bald heads. Some choose to cover their heads for religious reasons. And that is, and should be, just as acceptable as total baldness. During NAAF conferences there is complete acceptance of individual feelings and choices. There is no pressure on anyone to do anything that is uncomfortable for them; but there is complete freedom and support for those women and children who choose to be boldly bald. There is such joy in that freedom.

The 2010 conference had approximately 700 attendees including people with alopecia, their family members, spouses and friends. Some participants could only attend because of scholarships generously provided by the Foundation. There were bald heads everywhere, on people of all ages, sizes, shapes, colors, and gender. The hidden had become the norm. This three-day conference is, for some women, the only place they feel free to roam about without head coverings. I felt alive and energized, giddy and normal. Bald heads bobbing down the corridors, shining boldly through the glass elevator doors, and bedecking the escalators connecting the conference areas. And laughter, so much easy, happy laughter.

And the restaurant game? Well, to be perfectly honest, I was so busy meeting and greeting the bald women, men and children attending the conference, enjoying the company and the food , I forgot to count bald heads.

BOLDLY BALD WOMEN

There is something for everyone at the NAAF annual conferences.

• General information sessions and inspirational speakers set the tone, such as Kayla Martell, who did not allow alopecia to stop her from competing for—and winning!—the title of Miss Delaware 2010. Kayla went on to place in the top ten in Miss America 2011.

• A panel of experts discuss the latest advancements in understanding the 'hows and whys' of alopecia to answer on-going questions about alopecia areata.

• Workshops abound: for parents of children and pre-teens with alopecia, for young adults under the age of thirty, for women, men, for those without alopecia who want to support family or friends dealing with alopecia, and for those who want to learn how to apply makeup or choose and care for a wig.

• Trusted vendors are available to demonstrate and sell products and supplies for those interested.

• Throughout the conference, "camps" are simultaneously running for kids ages 5-10, tweens ages 11-13, teens ages 14-17, as well as meet-and-greets for the 18-24 year olds and another for the rest of the adults.

• There are activities to increase community awareness, and NAAF's premier fundraiser: The Tortoise & Hair™ Walk.

• Saturday night there is a dance for everyone and a dance contest for those who choose to participate with winners announced at the closing ceremonies on Sunday.

• Then comes the final farewell with light refreshments and time for last hugs and exchanges of phone numbers, email addresses, and ideas for next year's conference.

BOLDLY BALD WOMEN

When it's time to leave, each participant takes home the memories of good times, the knowledge that there is room for all, there is work to be done, and everyone can help. We can all become empowered to make a difference.

Thank you, NAAF, for all the workers and volunteers who make this powerful event happen year after year, and to all the generous contributors whose donations make NAAF's work possible. You are an unfailing light from which many candles are lit and glow forth with confidence and hope.

CHAPTER 9

Trichotillowhat?
There Is More Than One Road to Bald

⌒∽⌒

We can let circumstances rule us, or we can take charge
and rule our lives from within.
—Earl Nightengale

⌒∽⌒

That would be trichotillomania. It comes from the Greek words for 'hair pulling madness.' There are more reasons than alopecia and cancer for hair loss. Among them are:

- a malfunctioning thyroid gland
- hormonal changes due to pregnancy
- childbirth
- medications used to treat arthritis, depression, heart problems and high blood pressure
- discontinuation of birth control pills
- the onset of menopause
- physical or emotional shock such as the death of a loved one, trauma from a severe accident, surgery, sudden or excessive weight loss or a high fever
- hair styles that pull the hair too tightly as in pigtails or cornrows

BOLDLY BALD WOMEN

- scalp infections such as ringworm
- diseases that can cause scaring, such as lichen planus and some types of lupus
- trichotillomania

Trichotillomania is a form of traumatic alopecia. It is a compulsive disorder resulting in alopecia from repetitive hair manipulations and pulling as a means to relieve stress. It is more common in children and adolescents than in adults, and more common in female adolescents and adults than in male adolescents and adults. The hair pulling in trichotillomania is automatic, nonintentional, and mostly without any awareness of the repetitive twisting and pulling. It is estimated the number of people with trichotillomania is approximately five percent of the number of patients with alopecia areata.

Kathy Rymes contacted me asking if she could share the story of her experience with trichotillomania. She said, "If sharing it helps anyone, I am thrilled to have written it. As I continue on this journey, I cannot believe where I am today. Amazingly, I find myself starting to think that perhaps this long and difficult journey will have been worthwhile, will have served a purpose. If I can help anyone, anyone at all with their journey, then I am beyond humbled."

I think you will agree with Kathy once you've read her story.

My Story

If anyone ever told me a year ago that I'd be sharing my story, writing these words, facing the world each day "Boldly Bald," I'd have told them they were nuts. You see, mine is a story that spans nearly four decades, and until quite recently, it was my "dirty little secret." I spent all of my adult life in shame and anxiety, fear and despair, becoming consumed by this secret of mine. I tell my story today because, by the

82

grace of God, I can. No more "dirty little secret" and no more angst and despair.

For over thirty-six years I have battled a condition called TRICHOTILLOMANIA (TTM). Unlike alopecia, where the hair simply falls out and may or may not grow back in, my hair was compulsively pulled by me, until I was left with increasing and significant baldness. TTM was not a condition known in the United States by the popular media until about 1989. And for me, this means that I struggled many years, too many years, truly believing that I was crazy. After all, who pulls out their own hair and cannot stop this behavior? I knew no one who had this condition. And, each and every doctor I've seen has eventually told me that there appears to be no known cause and no known cure for TTM.

My journey has included therapy of various types, hypnosis and several different medications. No matter what I did, or how hard I tried, this impulse was and is bigger than I am. Trips to the hairdresser were incredibly anxiety provoking. A walk in the wind risked my hair shifting to show the bald spots. A relaxing swim on a blistery hot day would cause my hair to mat down awkwardly and show my secret. Every minute of every day I fought this stupid behavior. And, every minute of every day I struggled with the feelings of shame, embarrassment and despair. Why, oh why, would anyone pull out her own hair and not be able to stop? And when I learned of another hair loss condition known as alopecia, I actually wished that that was the reason behind my baldness. At least this would give me a reason to stop blaming myself.

Perhaps with age comes wisdom, an ability to be less critical of oneself, and an opportunity to look at the world and see what really matters. So, when my best friend was diagnosed with breast cancer, and she was faced with the ravages of chemotherapy and inevitable hair loss, having hair suddenly seemed far less significant. I had no problem en-

visioning her as the beautiful, wonderful person she is, with or without hair. I guess you could call it one of those light bulb moments when it all finally makes sense. No, I'm never going to make sense of this TTM "thing," but I have devoted so much time and energy, angst and shame towards it. It's only HAIR! To make the decision to shave my head was, incredibly, one of the easiest and most freeing decisions I have ever made. I shaved my head several days before my friend was to lose her hair. For very different reasons we were bald together. And nearly a year later, she is happy, healthy and has a full head of gorgeous hair. Thank God she is healthy. And me? Well, I'm "Boldly Bald!"

I did the wig and/or hat thing for many months. I still needed to hide the truth and was quite timid about the reactions I might receive. Incredibly, though, I was to find an immense relief and joy in being bald. For me, the urges to pull stopped, and I was actually rid of the hideous demon that had haunted me these many years. And then, I heard of International Alopecia Day, when women from all over the world celebrate the day without the cover or disguise of wig, hat or scarf. Hundreds, maybe thousands of women go forth on this day, embracing their baldness and simply celebrating life. Count me in! I dared to go out, face the world, boldly bald. Not wanting to wait for the big day, I actually celebrated my own Alopecia Day two months earlier! Yes, I was nervous, but I decided that I need to celebrate life too, and all the blessings that surround me.

I decided a few months ago to share my new look with my co-workers. The response I received was simply amazing. After all the years of hiding my dirty little secret, I was overwhelmed by the love, support and enthusiasm I received. There absolutely are questions every day, and not just a few questions of concern. "Are you sick?" "Do you have cancer?" I'm thinking that I should wear a shirt that proudly states, "Not sick, just bald!" Imagine, too, that people tell me each and every day that I'm

84

beautiful! I didn't know that my smile could be so wide!

I know that some will still question and perhaps judge my appearance. It's taken me many years to be comfortable and to accept myself as I am, Boldly Bald!! Interestingly, I have found that some of the people closest to me have been a bit hesitant to embrace my bald look. My husband in particular has struggled with my new public look. He loves me and supports me like no one else in the world can, but he admits to being protective. He worries about what others might say or how they might treat me, and he fears that I will be hurt or looked upon as odd. But this wonderful man is also my biggest fan and cheerleader. As he has seen my confidence and sense of peace grow, he's been steadfastly by my side to love me and support me and celebrate with me. I would be remiss to leave out the other two cheerleaders who continue to give me unconditional love. They, too, have learned to celebrate my beautiful bald look. My children have taught me that as long as I am okay with this look, they, too, will be okay. They tell me each and every day that they love me, that I'm beautiful and that they are proud to be my children. Surely, I am blessed.

It's been nearly ten months, since I shaved my head. I have never, for a single second regretted my decision. I've never felt beautiful, until now! I feel free and comfortable and blessed. I hold my head up high and find that with my self-assuredness and smile, I'm able to put most people at ease. The sight of a bald woman still causes a bit of concern, if not surprise, but I hope people will see us for the beautiful women we are. With all the goodness in the world, surely there is so much more to life than the stuff that covers our heads!

—Kathy Rymes

It is women like you, Kathy, women who have struggled to accept themselves and find inner peace and courage to be themselves, who teach the world every day that there IS so much more to life than the stuff that covers our heads.

CHAPTER 10

Yes, I Have No Hair Today...Maybe

⌘

*You have to accept whatever comes and the only important thing is
that you meet it with courage and with the best that you have to give.*
—Eleanor Roosevelt

⌘

This morning I made a cup of coffee, padded to the bathroom
to shower, and sang happily as the water bounced off my bald head.
When I'd finished showering, while brushing my teeth, I noticed a
few blemishes on my face.

Looking closer, the front lighting of the mirror and the back
lighting of the sun through the outside window merged, catching
patches of colorless strands on my face where the breakouts were.
HAIR! Not the fine, short, downy hair that used to cover my face,
but straggly goat beard hairs—the ones that had you grabbing for
the tweezers back when hair was not a novelty. But these hairs look
confused. They were the non-color of clear fishing line and had no
sense of uniformity at all!

The more I looked the more astounded I became. Nope, no
nose hair, but there were ridges growing along the outside edges of
my ears like transparent pine trees storming the heights of a barren
mountainside. No eyebrows, but a patch of hair wannabes at the nape
of my neck.

BOLDLY BALD WOMEN

This has happened before. In the past all the new hair quickly fell out again leaving me once more smooth as a baby's butt and blemish free. What will happen this time?

Alopecia is fickle. If you let it, it will indifferently drive you crazy. Just when you've given up all hope, hair will grow back, stay for a while, or maybe forever, and fall out someplace else—or not. And when you've finally dared to breathe a sigh of relief because it's all grown back and taken up permanent residence, whole communities just disappear, leaving bare patches of scalp behind like abandoned camp sites. Or it may all leave en mass, and you stand looking in the mirror at a totally new personal landscape, trying to see if you are still in there somewhere.

One of the difficult aspects of alopecia is that you don't get to grieve a loss, adjust to a change in your self-concept and physical appearance, and then move on with your life. It keeps you off balance and feeds both false hope and unfounded despair again, and again, and again, until the only thing you know for sure is nothing is for sure. And that certainty of uncertainty is called acceptance. It's a good place to be, and it's a hard place to remain centered.

For today, I feel okay about this new development, although honestly, I hope the little buggers decide to leave sooner rather than later. I've grown fond of my smooth skin and shining head.

Speaking of fickle...

This story comes from Karen Denfeld Adams. Karen turned on a light bulb of understanding over my shining head as to just exactly how unpredictable alopecia can be.

ൟ

BOLDLY BALD WOMEN

During the summer of 1983, I lost my first patch of hair. Since I had long hair, I hadn't even noticed it. A friend of mine spotted it when I bent down to pick something up. I thought it was strange, and I was obviously concerned when I actually felt my bald scalp for the first time. She suggested that I go see a dermatologist to find out why.

It was a little reassuring to me when I saw the doctor and he took one look at my bald patch and said, "Oh, that's just alopecia areata."

My reaction of course was something like, "What the heck is that?"

At that time it was widely thought that alopecia areata was caused by stress. I thought that was odd because I didn't feel like I was under any stress. I was home on summer break from college, working a part-time job and hanging out with my friends every chance I had. I was happy. When the doctor said there was a treatment for it, I got the cortisone injections in the patch, scheduled a follow-up appointment for the following month, and went on my way. When I went back the next month, the bald patch was gone, and I now had a patch of new hair in its place.

It was several years later before another bald patch appeared. By this time, I was out of college, but I went back to the same doctor to get my injections and went on with life. There was a shorter time frame between patches two and three, and so my concern grew as to what alopecia areata really was and where it might take me. I started questioning the doctor further about alopecia areata. He wasn't able to answer my questions to my satisfaction. I apologized to him, explaining that I was going to seek a second opinion. He understood and wished me well.

I found another dermatologist and made an appointment. I fell in love with him as soon as he walked in the exam room. It's hard to explain, but he just had a way of making you feel at ease and comfortable. He knew why I was there, because when I set up the appointment I told them why I needed to see the doctor. He immediately suggested that we should determine for sure if this was really alopecia areata by taking a

88

sample of my scalp and having the follicles looked at.

I had not been aware that this could be done and thought, yes, that way I would know for sure what I was dealing with. Maybe it wasn't alopecia areata. Maybe it was something else. The test came back that some of my follicles had the characteristics of alopecia areata. Deep down I knew this was true, so, it didn't come as any big surprise. Of course, my new doctor agreed with the first doctor that alopecia areata was caused by stress. This still baffled me, because I didn't feel like I was under any stress. I was in my early twenties, a college graduate with a job and lived in my own apartment. I tried to make a conscious effort to relax, but that began stressing me out, so I just forgot about it. I would receive my injections whenever a patch showed up. The hair always grew back, so it was no big deal. I just dealt with each patch as it came and continued on with my life.

This is how alopecia areata affected me for the first eleven or so years. I would get a patch, have it treated, the hair grew back. During this time, I went to the same beautician for my haircuts, perms, hi-lights etc. When I had hair, I definitely had fun with it and liked changing my style. Maybe deep down I knew I didn't have much time to enjoy it.

By the fall of 1994, I was married and my husband and I had been blessed with our second child that May. I was at the salon getting my hair cut to head back to my college to spend Homecoming weekend with my girlfriends. I was looking forward to a weekend of fun when my beautician told me I had another patch. I remember giggling and saying something like, "Here we go again."

It had been a while since my last patch and I had almost forgotten about alopecia areata (if you can believe that). This time, something was different though. When I went back for my follow-up a month after my injections, there was not any hair regrowth. The doctor gave me another round of injections and instructions to come back next month. During that month between follow-ups I realized how much hair I was losing. I had to gather up hair from my pillow each morning and clean out the drain at the end of my shower. For the first time, alopecia areata was affecting my life, and I wasn't having fun anymore. I began doing research as to what this condition really was and I learned a lot. When I went back for my next follow-up, I didn't need my doctor to tell me that there was no regrowth, I already knew because I had been looking for myself. I told my doctor about how much hair I was losing. I mentioned the research I had been doing about alopecia areata and that I didn't want to do the injections anymore because they were obviously not working. He agreed that was probably a good idea. I told him that I was just going to see where this journey was taking me and thanked him for all that he had done to help me over the years.

My hair was getting so thin by the spring of 1995, there was no hiding it anymore. My mom took me out and bought me my first wig. I hated it from the beginning, but I didn't want to make other people uncomfortable, so I wore it.

Can you believe that? What was I thinking? I would wear my wig to work, sit at my desk all day while my hair fell out from under the wig. Then, as soon as I walked thru my front door, I took off the wig and tried not to feel sorry for myself. It was tough at times, and the tears did come, but only when I was home in my room. I didn't want anyone to feel sorry for me, so I hid myself away when things got too hard and I had to let it out.

One evening during one of these difficult times, my husband came to me and said, "Why don't we just shave it all off?"

I looked at him like he was crazy. Was he kidding? Shave off what little hair I had? How could he even suggest that to me? He pointed out to me that he didn't marry me for my hair, and since it was falling out a little more each day, why not just get rid of it all at once, and be done with it? So, there I sat in the bathroom, while my husband cut my hair to the scalp. Then he took a razor and shaved it clean.

It was liberating! I felt like I had beaten alopecia areata. It couldn't do anything to me anymore because I got rid of everything it was taking away from me. The next morning when I woke up, I turned to gather the hair off my pillow and realized I didn't have to do that anymore!

Instead of my wig that day, I put a baseball cap on my head and walked out the door. Why not? My husband had just told me how beautiful I was without hair and his opinion was the only one that mattered to me. Why did I have to worry about how other people felt? I became a different person, more confident. My husband told me that I was meant to be bald because I had a perfectly shaped head. People started telling me how beautiful my eyes were, that they had never really noticed them before. Of course, the baseball cap was my security blanket. If I walked out the front door, I had to have it on my head. I knew I wasn't hiding the fact I was bald, but I wasn't ready to show off my baldness to the outside world just yet. I wore hats and scarves in my day-to-day life in the beginning. I even wore the wig occasionally because, for some reason, I felt there were some places that I should wear hair.

At the end of 1997, I found out I was pregnant with our third child. This would be the first pregnancy for me as a bald woman. How would people react when they saw a bald pregnant woman, because of course, most people thought I had cancer when they saw me. What would their reactions be? Believe it or not, my hair started growing back. Of course, it was a totally different color than what my natural hair color had always been. My hair was always a shade of light brown, but when it came back in during the pregnancy, it was jet black.

By the end of the pregnancy I had enough hair that I had to get it cut. This was a strange new world for me. It hadn't been that long, but I had already forgotten what it was like to have to wash and style my hair in the morning. I wasn't sure if I liked having to do this again. It took

BOLDLY BALD WOMEN

away time I needed to take care of my three kids before walking out the door each morning.

About nine months after the birth of our third child, I was starting to get used to this new routine. Then I realized that I was gathering hair off my pillow in the morning and cleaning out the drain after my shower again. I knew what was coming. It was inevitable. I shaved off my hair a few weeks later. I left my life with hair again and returned to my life with alopecia areata. It was so familiar to me, I didn't really skip a beat. My children knew me as a bald mom. My baldness was familiar to them too. So, I pulled my hats, scarves—and even the wig—out of storage, and began to wear them again. The wig was the first item to make it back to the closet. I hated it from the beginning, but when there was no hair on my head again I realized how uncomfortable it was on my bare scalp. I was done with it for good! I continued with the hats and scarves. Occasionally, I ventured out without anything on my head. When I did that, I felt like a rebel. I had seen other women do this, so why couldn't I?

It was fun feeling that freedom, but the next day I would always find myself reaching for a hat. It was June of 2010 when I shed my hats and scarves for good. It was a brutally hot Virginia June, and I was waiting for my oldest son's high school graduation to begin. A black woman sat down in front of my husband and me with her hair shaved so close to her scalp she might as well have been bald. We greeted each other as she sat down. She was beautiful. I looked at my husband and smiled thinking, "Why don't I have the guts to do that?"

At the end of the graduation when we walked out of the air-conditioned building into the oppressive 100+ degree day, the scarf on my head felt very uncomfortable. We snapped a few pictures and we all agreed to head down the road to our favorite local Italian restaurant for a celebratory graduation lunch. In the car on the way there, I pulled my scarf off to allow my head some fresh air and mumbled something about having to put it back on. My husband said, "Why?" and that was the

92

last time I wore anything on my head. Now, if I do wear a hat or a scarf, it's as an accessory not a necessity.

I began a new journey on June 5, 2010. I'm not saying I don't still have my bad days, because I do. I know I'm always going to cross paths with the occasional person who doesn't know how to deal with someone who is different. But those times are outnumbered by the people whose lives I touch in a positive way. A couple of years ago, I was shopping at Target and realized I kept crossing paths with a young woman in her early twenties. I wondered why she kept popping up where I was in the store, and then she approached me.

I knew what was coming. She thought I had cancer and wanted to talk to me. She had just been diagnosed and was told she was going to have chemotherapy. She had long hair and was terrified to lose it. I told her my story in the short time we had standing there in the middle of the store, explaining why I had chosen not to wear a wig. Before I knew it she was squeezing my hand and saying, "Thank you, I'm not afraid anymore."

I recently happened to get in the line of one particular cashier at my local grocery store who, as she rang up my sale, asked me why I was bald. I told her my story. She got excited, saying that she had alopecia too, but was afraid to go without her wig.

She said, "I really hate my wig, and when I go home tonight, I'm going to shave off the little bit of hair I have left and shed my wig too."

Now, she is a proud, bald woman too! These are just two times out of many that I have crossed paths with someone who has said that I've helped them in some way. What they don't realize is that they have helped me too. It gives meaning to the question of why God blessed me with alopecia areata.

—*Karen Denfeld Adams*

BOLDLY BALD WOMEN

⮞⮜

Ahhh, do you see? Karen has found a way to not only accept alopecia, but to embrace it as the blessing it can be. Her husband, like my little Greek, was her mainstay and wellspring of daring. Look what his encouragement for his wife did to help two women he never met deal with their fear and unwarranted shame!

Karen's story clearly delineates one of the ways this autoimmune disorder works. It shows, once again, that uncertainty is the only certainty of living with alopecia. What I love best about Karen's story is the powerful demonstration of potential good it conveys. Each woman who chooses to walk the boldly bald path has the potential to touch and inspire others, both with, and without hair, male and female alike. It is truly a domino affect, like one of those exhibitions where thousands upon thousands of dominos have been set up to initiate chain reactions. Every domino affects every other domino. The end result is a wonder of design and precision. I believe that is how God works in our lives. We each touch another, who touches another, who touches another, until God's design for our lives is complete. Sharing our stories is the precipitating action that leads to a change of society's perception of female baldness.

Karen's own research, her decision not to endure painful treatments, but to follow the journey to see where it took her was the first domino. Her husband, her wonderful angel of a husband, was the second domino. His response was about as perfect a response as ever could be hoped for. His love, and the reassurance that he didn't marry her for her hair, gave Karen a solid base upon which to build self-confidence. His shaving of her head was an act of loving acceptance and active support. It was proof positive of the authenticity of his active partnership in Karen's venture into baldness.

The third domino was the comments of friends and acquaintances telling her how beautiful her eyes are. They noticed, and reacted to, what was there rather than what was missing.

Then there was the woman who sat in front of Karen at the graduation ceremony that hot Virginia June. It was just a simple greeting, an acknowledgement between two women. Did the woman with her hair shaved close to her scalp have any idea of what her choice had sparked? Who knows? But, she was the fourth and final domino in the chain of events that led Karen to go publicly boldly bald.

Did the chain reaction stop there? Of course, it didn't. The ripples continue throughout the world even now.

Do you still think you are insignificant, and your decision whether to take the boldly bald path or not doesn't matter? Think again.

৵৽৵

P.S. To husbands, significant others, fathers, sons, grandsons, nephews and anybody else with 'Y' chromosomes I may have missed, when you throw a stone of support into the pond of female baldness—whatever the reason for hair loss—you cannot imagine the extent and effect of your caring action. What you do, or don't do is crucial to how well the women in your lives cope with hair loss. Keep reading, you get a whole section to yourselves later in this book in the *Notes From Alopecians* chapter.

CHAPTER 11

CHAMPIONS

෨ඁ෨

*There is no passion to be found playing small—in settling for a life
that is less than the one you are capable of living*
—Nelson Mandela

෨ඁ෨

There are two meanings for the word champion. The first is:
One that holds first place or wins first prize in a contest.

As I write today, I'm thinking about the recent Olympic Games.
Champions who made it to the podium were on the minds of the
millions of people around the world who avidly followed the games.
What a ride it was. Swimmer, Michael Phelps, became the most deco-
rated Olympian in history with twenty-two medals.

Then there is Gabby Douglas, who at sixteen years old was the
first African American to win the title of best all-around gymnast.
While Gabby was busy winning gold, a few bystanders complained
her hair was out of order and needed more attention. Really? She is
vaulting and swinging and tumbling and flying through the air prov-
ing she's the best gymnast in the world and hair still takes priority?

How about Oscar Pistorious, twenty-five, of South Africa,
nicknamed Blade Runner? He came in dead last in the 400-meter
semi-final individual running race with a time of 46.54 seconds, but

could not advance to the finals. Grenadian, Kirani James won the gold medal in the final event with a personal best time of 43.94 seconds—a whopping 2.6 seconds between Pistorious not running in the finals and James's gold medal. Did I mention Pistorious was born without fibulas and had both legs amputated below the knee when he was eleven months old? Pistorious ran the race on carbon fiber blade prosthetics. Some folks were worried artificial legs gave him an unfair advantage. Let's see, no legs in prosthetics versus two real legs with trained muscle and sinew. Yeah, sure, a big advantage goes to the guy with no legs pounding his stumps into the receptacle on top of his carbon fiber blades. Pistorious' accomplishment was nothing short of astonishing.

Finally, we have twenty-three-year-old Joanna Rowsell of Great Britain. Joanna is one of a trio of Great Britain cyclists taking gold in the Women's Team Pursuit event. What's so special about Joanna? She stepped onto the podium to receive her gold medal without her wig, thus exposing her bald head to the world. Joanna has had alopecia areata since she was ten, but she refused to allow it to take over her life and diminish her determination to race. Rowsell spoke with the Daily Mail about her alopecia: "I was gutted when it happened. I had been a girl who loved having my long hair in plaits. I remember crying one night to my parents and asking why it was happening. They said they would find someone to fix it."

Of course, her parents couldn't find someone to fix Joanna's alopecia. As yet, there is no cure. She went on to express the difficulty of being a teenager with alopecia. She didn't bother with make-up or clothing because she didn't want to think about her appearance. When she was fifteen, Joanna was spotted by British Cycling's talent scouts. She won the Junior Women's National 2K Individual Pursuit title and kept right on cycling to Olympic gold.

BOLDLY BALD WOMEN

"Now," she says, "I cannot imagine my life if I had not had alopecia. I don't know what route I would have taken. It scares me to think I would not have found cycling. The alopecia made me very shy so I stayed in and intensely focused on my homework or that 'A' in an exam. Working hard was the only thing that stopped me from worrying about the future, about whether I would get a boyfriend or how I would face getting a job with strangers.

"Then cycling came along and I applied the same work ethic. I worked through any worries I had about my hair and I focused solely on cycling. It made me who I am."

CHAMPIONS OF BALD

The second definition of champion is: *One who fights for or defends a cause or another person.*

Joanna Rowsell is not only an Olympic Champion, she is a Champion of Bald. Joanna's courage shows female baldness does not have to be synonymous with sickness or shame. Standing boldly bald in front of the millions of people watching around the world brought awareness to alopecia. Awareness sparks curiosity. Curiosity enables education. Education is the precursor to change in attitudes and actions towards all bald women, regardless of the reason for their baldness. Joanna said: "I got a tweet this morning telling me that it was International Alopecia Day and I thought it was a bit spooky that it fell on the same day as our final. If I can help people with alopecia then that is great—it is good to be able to raise awareness of it."

Boldly Bald is not the end of big dreams.

Kayla Martell, crowned Miss Delaware of 2010, began to lose her hair when she was only ten, but that didn't stop her from dreaming about being on the Miss America stage. She has competed both with and without wigs. During an interview on CBS's *The Early Show*, Kayla said it was not in spite of alopecia, but because of it that she wanted to compete in the pageants. "I knew that I had to be on Miss America's stage, and I had to get there somehow." Kayla believes she'd probably be a more effective beauty queen without wearing wigs. Her dream is to increase public awareness of alopecia. On her blog she writes, "I know in my heart that every girl is a beauty queen whether she has hair or not!" Kayla is another Champion of Bald.

Don't think for a moment becoming a Champion of Bald starts out on, or has to end up with, standing on a world-wide podium. It begins within each of us. Championship begins as a seed when we look with horror into the mirror and see the first bald patches. It is watered with shower spray mingled with tears as we look down to see the drain clogged with clumps of hair. It grows as we learn to accept ourselves as we are, and love ourselves, not in spite of hair loss, but because of the realization we are not our hair. It is fertilized with the unconditional love and support of significant people in our lives. Championship matures with the overcoming of the ridicule and prejudice we often face every day. And it bears fruit when we can see it as a blessing enabling us to become agents of change, whether that change is on a world wide, public podium or the relative obscurity of our individual lives.

Boldly Bald is not the end of your love life.

My name is Dotty, I'm 41 years old, I live in New Hampshire, USA, and I have had AU [autopecia universalis] for almost four years. I started to lose my hair in patches after a very traumatic experience. I suppose, in retrospect, losing all my hair is nothing compared to finding out that the man I married molested my daughter. I put the monster in jail, my daughter in therapy, and tried to be strong. I worked harder than ever to keep my girls happy, the house payments made, my bills paid, and my childcare center from going under with only one paycheck instead of two. I kept everything inside instead of asking for help.

I think my body fought me because it needed an out for all the bottled up stress. That's where the hair loss came into play. I noticed a few small patches of hair missing in the beginning of October in 2001. By the end of that October, the patches were increasing in size and quantity. By February of 2002, I had lost most of the hair on the top of my head. My hair was still pretty long in the back, so I was able to wear a bandana and still at least look normal to everyone else. But, waking up every morning with a pillow full of hair and gobs of my hair in the drain every time I took a shower was too much for me to take. I was even afraid to brush or comb my hair for fear of pulling the rest out! I finally decided it would be better for me to shave off what little hair I had left and wear a wig.

Well, my first couple of wigs ended up sailing across the room because I hated the way they looked on me. I didn't know that they could be thinned out to look more natural. It took me a few months to get used to wearing a wig and realizing that nobody was staring at me and noticing that I was wearing fake hair.

At that time I had been dating a man for about four years. He decided to wait until I was completely bald to tell me he didn't want to see me anymore. Of course, he said it had nothing to do with my hair. I was completely devastated to say the least. I was still having a tough time with my daughter. She was not doing well in school and was having major self-esteem issues. The excuse he used for leaving me was that I had too many problems in my life—meaning my daughter.

Okay, so there I was, a thirty-nine-and-a-half-year-old bald woman with a troubled child. Who the heck was going to want to deal with that? I went through the dating scene, telling the men up front

BOLDLY BALD WOMEN

about my hair loss. After all, I was dealing with it, and anyone I would get involved with would certainly have to deal with it too. Most of them would say it didn't bother them, but it really did, and I wouldn't get a call back. Until I met Brett.

I met him online (yes, really!) through a mutual friend. I made sure she told him about my bald head. He said, "Hair doesn't make a person," and he really meant it. He is a wonderful man who loves me for the person I am, not for my appearance. He loves my daughters like they were his own, and has accepted Kristin, problems and all. He has custody of his ten-year-old son. It has been two years since I met him. We married and are now all one big happy family all these years later.

~∞~

I met Dotty and Brett at a NAAF conference. My nickname for Brett is Scout, because he can find anything anyone needs in a strange city, and because he has a great sense of direction, whereas I can get lost in a paper bag with both ends open. Dotty and Scout bring joy and laughter wherever they go. They are two of the kindest, most caring people it has ever been my privilege to meet. All it takes is one look at the two of them together to know that Boldly Bald definitely does not mean the end of a healthy, happy and successful love life! Dotty is a champion. She is a champion of living a boldly bald life, a champion of dealing with the curve balls life can throw at us, and she is a champion of faith in herself and persistence. And Scout? Well, he's a champion of smart and good taste.

Boldly Bald is a life-line for others.

I met YoKasta at the same NAAF alopecia conference where I met Dotty and Brett. YoKasta has become comfortable with her baldness and confident within herself. Sometimes she simply glows. YoKasta shares this touching story about an interaction with a co-worker.

101

BOLDLY BALD WOMEN

On my new job, I'm the only woman in my department. How-ever, we share office space with the patient accounts people in one of the corporate headquarters buildings. At the end of my first week there, this beautiful lady came up to me with tears in her eyes and hugged me. It caught me off guard, so I asked her why she was doing so.

Her answer was this, 'God places people in other people's lives for a reason. I just started chemotherapy and radiation for ovarian cancer and I was told that I would start losing my hair within two weeks. I used to have really long hair, but now I've cut it into a pixie cut and I've been worried about how I'm going to look bald. I bought some scarves, but I don't want to wear them in the heat and I refuse to wear a wig. I was just praying and asking God to send me a sign that everything would be all right, and just as I looked up, I saw you walking toward your office. When I saw you, I just had to come and hug you. Thank you for showing me that if you can rock a bald head, then so can I.'

I told her that I had alopecia and not cancer, but she didn't care about WHY I was bald. Rather, she was concerned about having the confidence to be herself and having the courage to control what she could in facing what is truly the fight of her life.

Well, this wonderful woman came into work today with a beauti-ful bald head after shaving her head last night when her hair started coming out in clumps in the shower. The thought occurred to me as I was hugging her and sharing a couple of tears right along with her, that all too often we concern ourselves so much with what we think is wrong with ourselves, that we fail to see how much of an inspiration we can be to oth-ers, regardless of the reason for either their hair loss or ours.

I was genuinely humbled that this lady took the time to come to me and share her story, and even more so, considering that she is fifty-four years old—literally old enough to be my mother. The strength and courage that she has displayed thus far has inspired me and renewed my spirit, and serves to remind me—as it should remind all of us—that you just never know whose lives we touch simply by being ourselves. Don't sweat the person in the mirror or the voice in your head that tells you that your bald head doesn't do or bring anything positive in your life. I guarantee you that if you believe that, you're dead wrong!

YoKasta is a Champion of Bald. She is also a champion of empathy and compassion. YoKasta is helping to update the language of hair. She is redefining the definition of baldness from shameful and sickly to bold and beautiful. You go, YoKasta, you go!

⌒◦⌒

What makes you who you are? Do you allow baldness or the reactions of others to define your worth and value? Do you shrink from the world, or do you use alopecia as a means to grow courage and self-confidence, to increase public awareness, to educate, and to facilitate change in the perceptions of others towards female baldness?

The choice is yours. If you are caught up in the shock and grief of losing your hair, or are afraid of the reactions of others and just want to hide, please believe you are not alone. We have all been there. Some of us stayed there, thinking it to be the safer, less painful choice. More and more of us are coming to believe that hiding is, in fact, more damaging to our self-esteem and more painful than living openly with hair loss. More and more of us are reaching out and drawing strength and courage from each other. More and more of us are letting go of the angst of being different and replacing it with pride in ourselves and excitement about the potential for change we are privileged to be in a position to effect.

You, too, can be A Champion of Bald

If you so choose, you, too, can be a Champion of Bald whether on a world podium, or in the privacy of your own kitchen over a cup of coffee with a friend. Baby steps, dear hearts, baby steps will take you wherever your spirit leads you. Look to your deepest self to see the bald reflection in your own mirror with the same tenderness you would if someone you love had lost all of their hair. Love and accept yourself as you would love and accept them.

Share your condition with trusted family and friends and remember to give them time to process their initial reactions before you think you've read negativity into the looks on their faces. It takes each of us time to process our own first reactions to our hair loss. Others need processing time too. Most of all, it is your own attitude toward your baldness that has the biggest impact on others.

Get support from NAAF and Alopeciaworld.com. Both of those resources make great coaches. Get involved with International Alopecia Day. You might just be able to find someone else in your area who could use a friend who really understands.

Make a list of things that are great about being bald. Don't worry if you can't think of even one in the beginning. The list will come as you open your heart.

The more boldly bald women out in the world, the less of a novelty we will be, and the more people will become accustomed to seeing bald women on the streets. Buy yourself some kicky earrings to give your head pizzazz, and get out there and strut your stuff, if only out of the front door to get your mail.

Every champion starts at the first step and trains and practices all the way to the podium. You, too, are a champion, even if you don't know it yet.

CHAPTER 12

International Alopecia Day™—Mary Marshall's Story

಄෴

Your time is limited, so don't waste it living someone else's life. Don't be trapped by dogma—which is living with the results of other people's thinking. Don't let the noise of others' opinions drown out your own inner voice. And most important, have the courage to follow your heart and intuition. They somehow already know what you truly want to become. Everything else is secondary.
—Steve Jobs

಄෴

Mary Marshall is an unassuming woman of remarkable talents and undertakings. She is a former attorney turned folk dancer/ teacher and she is the drummer in two San Diego folk bands—Eastern Exposure and Dromia. Mary travels throughout the world with her husband, Steve Gould, who is a renowned landscape, nature, and underwater photographer. As Mary travels her own journey through alopecia, she has become a focal point of international notoriety as the creator and coordinator of International Alopecia Day™ (IAD).

IAD had humble beginnings as an opportunity for women with alopecia to experiment with going bald in public. As Mary tells us, IAD has grown to include gatherings of Alopecians—women, children and men—and their family and friends in many countries around the world.

Each year, everyone involved sends Mary pictures of their worldwide celebrations and Mary compiles the pictures into a video posted on YouTube. Mary's efforts have done much to increase alo-

BOLDLY BALD WOMEN

pecia awareness and promote self-acceptance and courage for women to go boldly bald into their lives. Here is her story.

಄

I was always proud of my beautiful, thick hair—waist-length and straight circa 1970, big and permed in the 1980's, and later a short professional cut. About thirteen years ago, when I was in my late forties, I had my first bald spot, which was diagnosed as alopecia areata. I was surprised, but not too worried, because the spots were small, infrequent, and not visible. It never occurred to me that I might go bald. Dermatologists injected cortisone into the bald spots periodically for seven years. Hair grew back in the areas of the injections, but often fell out again.

In 2007, the bald areas started to appear more frequently, and then they got bigger and merged. After a few months, the shots were no longer an option because the bald areas were too large. I took Prednisone for one month when the hair loss accelerated, but it had no effect. I became very depressed, cried a lot, and constantly checked my head for expansion of the bald areas. I finally took charge and shaved my head in January 2008, and immediately felt better! Shaving gave me control again. I stopped worrying about losing my hair once it was all gone. I emailed photos of the "new me" to my friends and relatives.

By three months later, I had no hair on my head—alopecia totalis. I was happy that at least I still had my prominent eyebrows and lashes. But, by May 2008, I had lost every hair on my body and progressed to alopecia universalis. Since then, I've twice had my eyebrows, eyelashes, nose hair, and facial peach fuzz grow back for a number of months, only to fall out again. It's difficult when this happens, but these days I try not to get too emotionally attached to my eyebrows if they grow back. I've had permanent makeup (tattoos) eyebrows and eyeliner since 2008, and it works well for me.

106

BOLDLY BALD WOMEN

I don't believe that anything happened which triggered my hair loss. My best guess is that the onset of menopause and hormonal changes associated with it triggered the loss. To my knowledge, no one in my family has had alopecia areata. The doctors I saw didn't seem to know much about this disease. I think the most helpful thing I could've heard from my physicians would have been, "There is no cure for what you have, and no way to predict the course."

I bought my first wig before shaving my head. I had a very positive attitude about wigs and thought it would be fun to have lots of different hairstyles. I bought synthetic wigs and human hair wigs, but after about nine months of trying to wear them, I gave up. I eventually gave all my wigs away, and I don't think I'll ever wear one again. I'm happy for the women who can wear them, but for me, they were simply too uncomfortable and way too hot.

Not long after I lost all my hair, I was wearing a wig in a crowded theater without air-conditioning during a heat wave. Audience members were fanning themselves, waiting for a show to start. Sweat ran down my face and I thought I was going to explode from the heat building up in my body. Finally, I tore the wig off my head and threw it to the floor, shouted "F%#&!", and then started to cry. I was ashamed of my bald head, but couldn't stand the wig a moment longer. That was when I knew I had to find another solution.

I developed a way of wearing a particular kind of scarf, a Turkish scarf, and later made a video ("Alternatives to Wearing a Wig") about it, and put it on YouTube in August 2008 to help other women. I slowly started going out in public bald—a process that I called "'baby steps.'" For a long time, I kept track in a journal of my firsts—the first time I went to the mailbox bald, the first time to the grocery store, to the library, etc. Pretty soon I didn't need to keep track any more—it just became normal to be bald in public. And, I found that when I stopped being self-conscious and stopped thinking everyone was looking at me, it really seemed as if people weren't paying so much attention to my head. These days, I go bald everywhere, and only wear a scarf or knit cap when I'm chilly, or a hat when I need protection from the sun.

Even though being a bald woman is normal for me now, I'm frequently reminded that I look unusual when people mistake me for a cancer patient. When that happens, I'm polite and I explain about alopecia areata. Still, the cancer question does snap me back into awareness of my baldness at times when I've successfully forgotten all about it.

One time, a man working out next to me at a health club asked, "Are you sick, or do you do that on purpose?" When I explained, he said I look beautiful and started to flirt until I told him my husband likes my look (I had taken off my wedding ring to lift weights.) A woman I didn't know at the health club gave me a lovely necklace because she thought I was brave.

Only a few people have been rude or insensitive. One man in a waiting room just kept staring at me. Instead of looking away and ignoring it, as I usually do when people stare, I looked him in the eye and said, "Yes, I'm bald!" When he kept staring, I repeated the same thing louder. Then he came over to me and mumbled something about wondering why I shaved my head. Once at the zoo, a young boy pointed at me and shouted: "Mommy, that lady doesn't have any hair!"

In 2010, I was vacationing in Indonesia and had some very unpleasant experiences as a bald woman. With high heat and humidity, I didn't cover my head, and I got very different reactions to my baldness than I'd had in the States. Men would stop on the street, point at me and shout, "Why you cut your hair?" Or, they'd approach me in shops or other public places to ask me why I shaved my head. Many of them seemed outraged that I would make this choice. I learned how to say in Indonesian, "I'm sick. I don't have any hair." Near the end of the trip,

BOLDLY BALD WOMEN

I had the worst experience when some women at an airport began to laugh and point at me, and take pictures. They even came up and posed for photos next to me. It was awful.

There are also positive sides to my hair loss. I have super-smooth legs that I never have to shave. I can be ready to leave the house amazingly quickly. When I'm scuba diving, my wetsuit pops over my bald head much more easily, and after a dive, while everyone else has cold, wet hair, I'm completely dry in seconds!

I have had to let go of my previous notions of vanity and self-consciousness. I have come to a place where I mostly don't care what people think. I have learned that I'm stronger than I thought I was. I know I stand out in a crowd, and much of the time I feel exotic, special and beautiful as a bald woman. And, my collection of earrings has grown tremendously.

One relative refused to look at the bald photos and videos of me that I emailed to extended family members and friends. Finally, I confronted him in a telephone conversation, and told him how unsupportive I felt he'd been. It turned out that he thought I was militantly refusing to wear a wig. I explained about the excess heat of wigs, and he related to that immediately, since he also has problems with warm temperatures. I also told him that he needs to understand that this is a disease that I have no choice about, and I asked him whether he'd prefer I were terminally ill with cancer, or in a wheelchair with a disabling degenerative disease instead of only being hairless. Today, he is wonderfully supportive and has accepted me as I am.

My husband has been completely supportive from the beginning. He accompanied me to the hair salon for the initial shaving. He even offered to shave his own head! He encouraged me to go out in public bald if I would be more comfortable that way. I was self-conscious around him at first, but in a fairly short period of time, I began to believe what he was telling me,—that he still thinks I'm beautiful and that my bald-ness doesn't put him off.

I would advise family members of women newly diagnosed with alopecia, that—even when you think you've said enough positive things,—SAY THEM AGAIN! Keep telling her she's beautiful and that you love her. I'd also like people to know that it's okay to ask a bald person about their lack of hair. I prefer that people know I don't have cancer, rather than simply making the assumption that I do.

Helping other women who have alopecia has been of great help to me. Since 2008, I've been posting videos of myself online to show women that it's possible to be bald in public. I connected with women via the wonderful online community, Alopecia World, and made many Alope-cian friends across the United States and in other countries. Via Alo-pecia World, I've posted blogs and photos and responded to blogs posted by others. Now, through Facebook, I'm meeting and sharing with even more Alopecians around the world.

And, I created an international holiday, "International Alopecia Day™," now being celebrated all over the world on the first Saturday of August each year. My original idea was that for one day, women who've lost their hair could give going out bald in public a try. The holiday has evolved into a day for gatherings—large and small—of anyone, female or male, of any age who has alopecia, their families, and their friends. The goal is to take pride in who we are, have fun, and raise public aware-ness about alopecia.

The first International Alopecia Day™ took place in 2010. There are IAD groups on Alopecia World and Facebook. People send me photos of themselves taken on International Alopecia Day™ from where they live, and I create a YouTube video slide show of all the celebrations each year. In addition to many cities around the United States, countries that have participated include: The United Kingdom, Canada, Japan, Iran, Spain, Australia, France, Germany, and the Netherlands. The

BOLDLY BALD WOMEN

videos can be found on YouTube by searching for "International Alopecia Day". I hope to see the event grow each year to include more and more global locations.

For me, there is simply no other answer but to accept this new face I see in the mirror, be as healthy and strong as I can, and get on with my life! I believe bald women can change social attitudes and perceptions simply by going OUT. I feel strongly that this is an issue of equal rights: men with hair loss shave their heads, bald men appear in fashion ads and star in movies, people don't assume that bald men have cancer, and no one stares at a man because he's bald. I totally support women who prefer to wear wigs, but I want women to have the same option to go bald in public that men do, and not be forced to endure head coverings if they find them uncomfortable or hot.

My greatest hope is that bald women in public will one day become as unremarkable as bald men. I don't expect this to happen in my lifetime, but things are already changing as more and more women opt for freedom and comfort.

Oh, Mary! You and I share the same hope. And things are changing—more quickly than I had ever imagined. It seems acceptance of female baldness is growing exponentially as the word spreads and more and more courageous women choose to accept and love their beautiful bald heads and to stand above the crowd with confidence and pride.

CHAPTER 13
And a Child Shall Lead Them

৵৵

If your actions inspire others to dream more,
learn more, do more and become more, you are a leader.
—John Quincy Adams

৵৵

Olivia. Dear, amazing, most atypical of typical teenagers, nonchalant, straight up, fun and funny Olivia. What can I tell you about Olivia?

I met Olivia and her mother, Sandy, at the 2010 NAAF Conference in Indianapolis, Indiana. The acceptance and hope at that conference completely blew me away, but not more so than my meeting with Olivia and Sandy. They touched me deeply. Their stories and antics left me breathless in shared laughter. Olivia modeled a pair of earrings my friend, Joyce, and I had developed as a prototype of the line of Boldly Bald Jewelry. Olivia modeled them stylishly. I remember thinking she was simply exquisite and hair would have somehow diminished her aura of playful light and grace.

And Sandy? Sandy is what every parent wishes their child would want them to be. Sandy, like every mom, wanted only the best for her daughter. She thought hair was the best, until Olivia told her otherwise. Sandy came to the realization that Olivia's best was different from what Sandy thought it should be. She made the decision to put aside her perspectives and support Olivia where she was, as she was. It was a courageous and selfless choice that opened the door to adventures and a platform where Olivia has been able to reach many children in ways neither Sandy nor Olivia could imagine.

Here is their story as it stands of this writing. I am certain we will be hearing a lot more about Olivia and Sandy in the years to come.

❧❧

SANDY:
THE TWO MINUTE CONVERSATION WITH
A STRANGER THAT CHANGED EVERYTHING

As I sat on the side lines that day at Conseco Field House, I watched my fourteen-year-old daughter, Olivia, get up and take the microphone. She had been asked to share her story with approximately 2,000 kids from Central Indiana, during The Choices for Champions Anti-Bullying Event. She walked with confidence and looked so cute, in what she called her "power outfit." It was a dress with a little black jacket and pink suede heels. Olivia appeared mature and older than her age. She spoke with ease and really held the attention of the audience. I was so proud of the way she inspired everyone who heard her speak. Sitting there, tearing up with pride, I reflected on everything that has happened to Olivia. Again, I marveled at the fact that all of her accomplishments may not have happened, if I had not had a two minute conversation with a stranger, when she was ten years old.

I remembered sitting in the nail salon, four years earlier. I could see Olivia with her nail technician getting her nails done, too. She loved this rare treat of mother-daughter mani-pedis. At ten years old Olivia was like most girls her age, she did well in school, had lots of friends and had recently discovered make-up. However, there was one very visible difference. Olivia was totally bald due to the medical condition alopecia. It had been about a year since Olivia shed her custom wig and bravely marched into her third grade classroom without hair.

I remembered watching her laugh and chat, very comfortable and confident. I, on the other hand, was on edge, as usual. Since Olivia would not even wear a hat on her head, we were approached often with carefully worded questions about Olivia's health. Obviously, everyone assumed she was going through cancer treatment. People were always kind and wanted to offer support. Most had gone through cancer themselves and wanted to share their stories. I was not upset by their questions, but when I saw someone watching Olivia, I was unsure if I should bring up her condition or wait for them to ask me. That day was no different.

While sitting under the hand dryer, a lady sat down beside me to dry her nails. She smiled and glanced at Olivia. Oh, no, here it comes, I thought.

The stranger asked, "Excuse me, is that your teenage daughter over there?"

I wasn't really up for the conversation, but she looked kind and smiled again, so I said, "Yes, that's my daughter Olivia, though she is not a teenager yet. She is only ten."

Then the woman surprised me with, "Can I tell you how beautiful I think she is? I have not been able to take my eyes off her since you arrived. She carries herself so well and she has such a style about her. I just had to tell you that I think she is so beautiful."

Wow, I was so touched. As any proud mom would, I said, "Thank you, so much!" Soon after, I paid the bill and we went about our day.

It wasn't until a few days later that the impact of our conversa-

tion fully hit me. The stranger had never even mentioned Olivia's lack of hair. She had actually commented on Olivia's beauty and saw that Olivia was uniquely pretty without hair. This amazed me. We had dealt with Olivia's alopecia for the past eight years, but nothing like this had happened before. WOW, this changed everything. All of the uncertainty that I had felt began to vanish. Could it be that all of my concerns about Olivia's hair loss and how people would respond to her could be unfounded? Could people really see her beauty the way I saw it? Was it really possible? This was just the shift in mind set that I needed.

You see, I am a single mom and Olivia is my only child. I did not have her until I was almost forty and she was my world. Though she was born five weeks early, Olivia was a healthy, normal baby. I loved being a mom and I really enjoyed dressing her up in cute little outfits. Everyone teased me about the fact that she was always so color coordinated, with lots of little accessories. I provided Olivia with bibs, pacifiers, socks and baby sunglasses in every color. One of my favorite memories was taking her to the mall and pushing her around in her stroller. Forty years of pent-up motherhood was pouring out on this one little baby girl, and I loved it. It was so much fun.

Everything felt perfect, until Olivia was eighteen months old. She was so cute with hazel eyes and a full head of blonde baby hair. On July 3, 1998, I had the day off from work, so I took Olivia for her first haircut at Cookie Cutters Haircuts for Kids. It was a really cute salon that catered to kids. There was an indoor playground and the styling chairs were kids sized cars, planes, horses and more. There were televisions at each station with movies and cartoons to choose from. Olivia was intrigued, but once the hair cut began, she got scared and began to struggle and cry.

As a memento of the first hair cut, we were given a lock of Olivia's hair, a photo and a certificate that stated, "Olivia has bravely submitted to the scissors of our stylist and completed all of the requirements of a first hair cut." It made me laugh, because it was so cute. I did not realize until later how valuable that little lock of hair would become to me.

Next, on our schedule that day, was Olivia's doctor's appointment for her routine vaccines. She cried there, too. It broke my heart to see her upset and we went home to recover from our rough day. It was Friday. By Monday, Olivia had a spot of hair loss the size of a quarter. Within days, her hair was coming out in handfuls. Obviously, I freaked out and rushed her back to her doctor. I was told that Olivia had developed alopecia, an autoimmune condition that causes hair loss. At the time, it affected over five million people in the United States. Though not life-threatening, it is a medical mystery and people affected by it can randomly lose, and re-grow, some, or all of their hair. Her doctor could not tell me if Olivia's hair loss would continue or if she would re-grow her hair. Unfortunately, within four weeks she was totally bald.

I was devastated and determined to find a cure, or at least more answers than I had. After several doctors and numerous types of treatments, we ended up at Riley Children's Hospital with Dr. Patricia Treadwell. Even though she was the top pediatric dermatologist, she had no more answers. She did, however prescribe a topical steroid and women's Rogaine. We began using it immediately and over the next several months Olivia's hair began to re-grow. By age four, Olivia had most of her hair back. I was thrilled and relieved! Now my daughter could start school and look like all of the other little girls. Because she was so young, I felt that she might not even remember being bald. She began school and everything was great.

My happiness lasted four years. During the summer when Olivia was eight, her hair loss began again. I was heart-broken! How would my little girl be able to handle this? Would she be bullied? What about when she was a teenager? Would this keep her from having a normal *life? How would boys react to it? I decided I would get the best wig on the market for her. I found a company in our area and discovered that a Custom Hair Systems wig would cost $6,000. I was a struggling single mom and that was totally out of my reach. I was, however, determined it was the right thing for my daughter. I negotiated a 'trade out' of services with the company and did marketing for them. Since they were new to our area, we allowed Olivia's story to be featured in the media. It was around the holidays and Stacia Matthews of WRTV TV, Channel 6, featured a story about Olivia receiving new hair for Christmas.*

When Olivia got her new hair, it looked amazing! Everyone loved it and no one was able to tell that she was bald. Unfortunately, it involved using a type of glue to attach the hair to Olivia's head. It was difficult, time consuming and itchy. Getting Olivia out the door for school became a huge challenge and most of the time, we were both in tears.

On one of these mornings, Olivia announced that she was going to school without hair. At that point, she had been wearing her wig for five months and the kids in her school had never seen her totally bald. I was sure this was a bad idea, but Olivia was adamant that this was what she wanted to do. Finally, I reluctantly agreed and we got to her school early so that I could speak to her teacher, the school nurse, the school counselor and the after school staff. All reassured me, and finally told me to go home, they would handle it.

So, at eight years of age, Olivia bravely marched into her third grade classroom without hair. I, on the other hand, sat in my car and cried like a baby.

Ironically, the teacher explained to the kids what Olivia's situation was and nothing bad happened. That day changed the entire direction of Olivia's life. Though I supported Olivia's decision, it was before I met the stranger in the nail salon. That two minute conversation helped me to understand what Olivia knew all along. Once Olivia and I were on the same page, everything changed.

117

BOLDLY BALD WOMEN

Soon after, Olivia and I founded Olivia's Cause. The purpose was to create awareness for alopecia. We wanted to help people going through what we went through. We started a support group and communicated with people from around the world about alopecia. We heard so many stories of people who were bullied, teased and even abused as a result of their hair loss. It affected us both deeply.

In 2008, we produced a music video about alopecia and bullying. Olivia starred in the video, playing the part of a teenage girl who was bald and being bullied. Her character went on to become a famous model and actress. The message was that you can be great, whatever your challenges are. We posted the video, "I Could Be Great," on You Tube and several other networking sites, with very positive feedback.

In May of 2008, Olivia was asked to share her story on Radio Disney's radio show, "Concerned Kids." At that point, her story had been featured in the media numerous times and she was very comfortable doing interviews. Olivia was a guest on the show and did a great job. This resulted in the offer of a job as a Kid Caster on the show. She began her professional career as an employee of ABC/Walt Disney at age eleven. She has worked for Radio Disney 98.3FM Indianapolis for the past three and a half years, and continues at the present time.

In addition, Olivia won the 2009 "Power of Children Award" from the Indianapolis Children's Museum where her story is on permanent display, the 2010 "Driven Like Danica Contest," from race driver Danica Patrick and the 2011 "Well Dunn Award" from Coach Lyn Dunn of The Indiana Fever.

In 2009, Olivia launched a lecture program where she began speaking to kids/teens in schools, churches and other organizations throughout Central Indiana. Her messages about it are that it is okay to be different, anti-bullying, teen suicide prevention, having self-confidence, and that you can be great, with or without hair. Olivia has spoken to literally thousands of kids/teens in schools and churches in these events. She has been praised by school administrators, principals, and teachers. Olivia is directly credited with influencing a boy in Franklin, Indiana, who planned to beat up another boy after school that day. During one of her appearances in Indianapolis, a young girl in the audience admitted that she had been considering suicide and changed her mind after hearing Olivia speak. Because she is making such an impression on her peer audiences, we have also published her story in a book called, Just Your Average Teenager Who Happens to Be Bald. The book, written completely by Olivia, has been distributed to 20,000 kids/teens through out Central Indiana and continues to sell as Olivia's story spreads.

Ironically, something that I thought would devastate our lives has brought some amazing opportunities to Olivia. I no longer worry about how Olivia will be treated by other kids or whether she will attend the prom or have boys like her. Everyone loves her. And she has NEVER been bullied. People ask us how Olivia can talk to other kids about bullying if she has never experienced it.

Her answer is, "Maybe kids have tried to bully me, but I am so confident, and because I handle it a certain way, bullying does not work on me."

As I watched Olivia finish her speech, my thoughts returned to the present moment. As usual, she asked if there were any questions. What happened next did not surprise me. Hundreds of kids began raising their hands to ask her questions. She handled their questions openly, honestly and humbly. Once again, she had inspired thousands of kids with her brave stance and ability to share her story. As the audience began to clap, I thought how far we had come since that day in the nail salon four years previously. I do not know the name of that stranger, nor would I recognize her if we met again. Still, I will never forget the two minute message she gave me and how it changed everything. For that I will be forever grateful.

BOLDLY BALD WOMEN

In January of 2012, Olivia and I were putting the final touches on her book, Just Your Average Teenager Who Happens to Be Bald. The Indianapolis Star Newspaper, that had done several stories on Olivia in the past, ran a feature about Olivia's new book. The story got picked up by USA Today, this resulted in a call from The Today Show. Olivia made an appearance with Kathy Lee and Hoda on February 28, 2012. Also, an online magazine in the UK picked up the story and as a result, Olivia was able to make an appearance on Elev8 TV show in Dublin, Ireland, via Skype. We receive orders for Olivia's book from all over the world.

In addition, Olivia was selected to receive "The Jefferson Award," a national award co-founded by Sam Beard and Jackie Kennedy. March of 2012, Olivia was selected as one of "The Pretty Amazing Girls of The Week" by Seventeen Magazine, and is currently featured on the Seventeen Magazine website.

Locally, Olivia continues to share her story with audiences as large as 2,000 kids and teens. With the help of sponsors, Olivia has been able to donate copies of her book to close to 4,000 kids who have heard her speak.

Please follow Olivia's Cause on Facebook. You can order her book at www.oliviascause.org

❧

OLIVIA:
I'M JUST YOUR AVERAGE TEENAGER
WHO HAPPENS TO BE BALD

"I don't know why kids listen to me, but they really seem to," Olivia writes. *"Maybe it is because I am their age, too, and I understand what they are going through in school. I am here to say I am just like you. I attend public school, I have to do homework, I hang out with*

my friends, I have sleepovers, I have to clean my room, and I am in the high school drum line. I am here to tell you that I am just your average teenager, who happens to be bald, and that you can be great no matter what you are facing. Everyone has it in them to do amazing things.

In my school they always say, 'Treat people the way you want to be treated...' When I look back and think about how many people suffer and are tortured just because they're considered different by society, it makes me realize that those words of wisdom are indeed so true."

❧

Olivia's message goes beyond encouraging bald children to accept themselves. It reaches beyond educating people about alopecia and helping to promote acceptance for children with alopecia. Her speeches encompass issues of insecurity and low self-esteem faced by most children and teens. She provides information about what bullying is, and what to do if you are experiencing bullying. She is concerned about teen suicide as a response to the stress of bullying in schools. Olivia counsels teens not to go down the suicide path, no matter what they are facing. She shares the effect her uncle's suicide had on her life as a way to help kids understand the impact of suicide on the lives of those left behind.

❧

"To this day," Olivia writes, "words can not describe how much I loved my uncle and how much he meant to me. When I share my message, I try to include how I felt about this because it brings a connection to me and kids who might be planning to commit suicide. The fact that I know how much pain his suicide brought to my life, I know how negative taking your own life can be."

❧

Olivia's mom, Sandy, points out that Olivia's alopecia, *"could have devastated her, but instead, it has given Olivia a powerful platform."*

BOLDLY BALD WOMEN

As of this writing, Olivia and Sandy have written a script for a movie presentation of Olivia's story and are looking at options to turn the project into reality to multiply the platform for Olivia's message a million-fold.

Olivia, like all teens, is busy trying on personas to see what fits and what doesn't. Her experiences with modeling and starring in a video have helped her to know she doesn't want to be either a model or an actress. But Olivia has a calling. She continues her public speaking and through it touches the lives of many, many, young people who will be the parents, family members, friends, classmates and co-workers, of the next generation. What Olivia says to today's children and teens will help determine tomorrow's attitudes and policies for the prevention of discrimination against bald women in society and the work place.

Olivia's words are changing the definition of beauty for an entire generation. Her belief that, *"You can be great, no matter what you are facing,"* is a catalyst for all who hear her to expand their thinking to acceptance of child and female baldness as just another normal facet of human physicality. I think we're going to see a lot more of Olivia in the years to come. That will indeed be a blessing.

CHAPTER 14

The Most Beautiful Flowers
Grow Out of the Deepest Piles of Shit

ೂೀ⊷ഏ

Consult not your fears but your hopes and your dreams. Think not about your frustrations, but about your unfulfilled potential. Concern yourself not with what you tried and failed in, but with what it is still possible for you to do.
—Pope John XXIII

ೂೀ⊷ഏ

Do you know how something inside recoils that first second after you say or do something your parents would have strongly disapproved of when you were a child? I got that internal reaction when I wrote the title for this chapter. I could hear my mother asking me if it was absolutely necessary to use the word 'shit.' In this case, Mom, yes it is. In this context the definition of shit is: a highly offensive term meaning to behave toward or criticize somebody with arrogant contempt and a total disregard for his or her feelings, especially from a position of power. And, the truth is, bald women are sometimes treated with contempt and a disregard for their feelings in the work place. That kind of treatment is highly offensive to women discriminated against because of their baldness. So, as the old saying goes, if the shoe (or in this case, shit) fits, wear it. What follows is a fictional story based on a composite of common experiences of women dealing with hair loss.

BOLDLY BALD WOMEN

Samantha loved flying. It was always an adventure to see who Fate would place in the seat next to her. Samantha sat in the aisle seat of the two-seat side section of the plane due to leave from San Diego. Given her Rubenesque figure, aisle seats were more comfortable. She hated the physical and emotional discomfort of climbing over someone on her way to the bathroom. She met the most interesting people on airplanes. This was the first time Samantha had flown without wearing a wig and she wondered what kind of response she would get from her seat mate. She looked up to see a petite brunette in business attire smiling in her direction.

"I believe my seat is the one next to you," the woman said. Her voice was rich and warm, her smile bright and genuine.

"Oh, of course," Samantha said. She stood, moving into the aisle for the woman to pass.

"Hi, my name is Desirae," the woman said as she settled into place and put her small carryon under the seat in front of her.

"Nice to meet you, Desirae, I'm Samantha. Where are you headed?"

"I'm going to Chicago for a business meeting, how about you?"

"I'm going to Washington, DC to a conference."

The two women chatted amicably while the plane taxied down the runway and lifted into the early morning sunlight. As the seatbelt sign blinked off, a blue eyed flight attendant with sleek black hair smoothed back into a tight knot leaned into the clanking stainless steel beverage cart that lumbered reluctantly down the aisle. "Would you care for something to drink?" she asked pleasantly.

"Coffee, please," Samantha said.

"I'll have the same," said Desirae, "and please keep it coming. It was an early morning and it will be a long, long day."

The stewardess chuckled, and said, "I understand completely

about long days," hoping soon she would get time for a cup of coffee for herself.

"So," Desirae said between sips, "what kind of conference is it?"

"It's an annual three-day conference put on by the National Alopecia Areata Foundation."

"I'm not familiar with that foundation. What do they do?"

"Well," Samantha said, searching for a starting point for her explanation, I have alopecia. It is an autoimmune disorder in which my body attacks my own hair. I have alopecia universalis—one of the most severe forms—which means all of my body hair has fallen out and, although the hair follicles are still present, my immune system won't let the hair grow again. There are a lot theories and suppositions, but nobody really knows why it happens. The foundation raises money for research into the cause and potential cures for alopecia, as well as education about the various kinds of alopecia, and provides support for everyone, including families, friends and co-workers of people dealing with hair loss due to alopecia. They also provide events to help raise global awareness for alopecia."

Samantha explained that the conference she was going to is held annually in different cities of the United States and that women, children and men from all over the world attend with their families and friends.

"What are the conferences like?" Desirae asked.

"They are so interesting and so much fun. The last one I went to had over 600 attendees, the majority of them were bald, although some wore wigs or head scarves. The hotel is taken over by bald," Samantha laughed, rubbing her head like a Buddha belly. "Suddenly, the haired folk are in the minority. It is fun to watch the wide-eyed bewilderment on their faces when they see so many bald heads in the hallways, jamming into the elevators and sitting in groups in the restaurants telling stories and laughing. Most wonderful of all is seeing the delight of the bald children as they see others just like themselves and get to feel part of the crowd. For some of them, it is the only time they go without some sort of head covering. During the conference they are just another kid playing with friends and participating in workshops."

She told Desirae of workshops for all ages and the events planned to raise awareness of alopecia in the host city. Samantha glowed as she spoke of the opportunities the conferences afforded Alopecians to teach other Alopecians. She shared her determination to do whatever she could to help make a place for bald women in a hair-addicted society—to change the perspective that female baldness is a sign of sickness and undesirability.

Desirae listened attentively as Samantha delineated NAAF's ongoing research into the cause and cure of alopecia. She sat spellbound as Samantha painted vivid word pictures of the suffering bald women and children face in a hair biased society.

"But your baldness doesn't seem to bother you at all. How is that?"

Samantha laughed heartily, her sea green eyes twinkling, and her long, gold earrings swinging in time with her laughter. "That's the me you see now," she said, her voice edged with irony. "Believe me, it's been a difficult struggle to get to this place of acceptance and gratitude."

"What happened?" Desirae asked, tipping her head to the right in an inquisitive gesture, her diamond earrings sparkling in the overhead light.

"Well, this happened quite a while ago. I wasn't looking for a job at that time. I was taking a sabbatical of sorts, staying home with my twins during the last summer before they left for college and before the empty nest syndrome would hit me head on. Once they left, I was casting about for something to fill the empty hours and help me reinvent myself after so many years of being a mom. A friend recommended me to a co-worker who was looking for help. The man called and asked me to come in for an interview. I thought it would be a step in the direction of finding something useful to do, so I agreed.

He said he was looking for a volunteer to help him in the office. I laughed and told him if he wanted me to volunteer, his work would be much lower on my priority list than if he paid me. He asked how much lower and I said somewhere after darning socks and before cleaning junk drawers. And I don't darn socks and rarely clean junk drawers."

Desirae chortled, exposing deep dimples in her cheeks. "Did he get your message?"

"Yep. After I told him my husband and I were supporting our twins through college, and I couldn't afford to give away my time at this phase in my life, he said he was certain he could fit a wage into his budget," Samantha said. "Seems he was just trying to get his work done without having to hit the company coffers. When he told me what he wanted, I made it clear some of his needs were within my skill set and experience, and some were outside my scope of reference. He assured me I would be trained for whatever I needed to learn. I guess he liked my personality and attitude. We agreed to give it a ninety-day trial and see where it led. I was surprised when a few people in the company wished me luck working for him. One, who had demanded a transfer back to her previous job after working for him only a few weeks, told me to watch out for his put downs and sarcasm. Really, Desirae, I couldn't imagine he could be so bad. He presented well, if a bit stiff in personality."

"Did you stay beyond the ninety days?"

BOLDLY BALD WOMEN

"Yes. At the end of the trial period, he wrote a glowing evaluation, gave me a raise and we agreed to make the part time job permanent. Slowly," Samantha went on, "his personality shifted. He became more demanding and intolerant. He gave one set of directions, and then, having forgotten what he said, confronted me for not doing the thing he thought he'd told me to do. When I tried to remind him he would sometimes stomp his foot and have a childish temper tantrum. Other times he would admit he had a problem with his memory and apologize."

"And you put up with that?" Desirae asked, her face contorted in disapproval. She stabbed at the call light. "Forget the coffee," she said. "This story calls for a drink. May I buy you one as well?"

Samantha snickered. "Much obliged. These memories leave a bad taste in my mouth."

When the stewardess arrived, Desirae said, "Two Jameson's on the rocks, please." She then looked at Samantha, who nodded her approval of Desire's taste in whisky with eyes twinkling. "Go on," Desirae said, "what happened after that?"

"My boss's behavior gradually became increasingly unprofessional. You asked me why I put up with it. Well, for one thing it was intermittent. We'd go for days or weeks with no problems and suddenly, without any reason I could discern, he would switch. One day, he directed a tantrum at me in the main office where others worked in crowded cubicles. I walked away, feeling embarrassed, humiliated and damn mad. I took the time I needed to calm down, then knocked on his door, entered his office and shut the door behind me. 'Nobody gets to speak to me that way, nobody.' I told him. I am your employee, not your whipping post. If you ever speak to me like that again, it will be the last time. I think from now on it would be better all around if you email me your instructions so neither one of us gets confused about them.' I walked back to my office, and closed the

128

door gently behind me."

"Did it get better?"

"For a while. We were in the middle of an important project, full of timelines and interactions with volunteer partners. Some of them flat out told me they would participate only if they could speak directly with me and not have to deal with my boss at all, which validated my belief that the problem was his, not mine. Stress began building up again—and my frustration right along with it.

"Why didn't you quit?" Desirae asked. She slurped an ice cube from the bottom of her plastic cup and chewed.

"I should have. I really should have, right then and there. But, despite the fact that my co-workers told me I was naïve and foolish, I still believed he could change for the better if I just held on long enough. Also, we were in the middle of that project and I didn't feel right about leaving him in the lurch."

"He didn't seem to have the same consideration for you," Desirae snorted.

"Seems that way, doesn't it? One morning when I woke up, I saw a clump of my curly, auburn hair on my pillow. I thought it odd, but shrugged and tossed it into the waste basket. When I showered, I looked down to see an enormous pile of soggy, tangled hair clogging the drain.

Over the next two months I lost every hair on my body. As the spots got larger, some people thought I was going through chemo. One woman in the company who knew very well what was going on in my office, put her hand on my shoulder and asked if I'd had enough of my boss yet."

The flight attendant passed their seats, a pillow and blanket in her arms. "May we have another round, please, when you have a moment?" Desirae said.

BOLDLY BALD WOMEN

The flight attendant smiled and nodded. "Of course," she said. I'll be right with you."

When she walked away, Desirae asked, "Do you hold your boss responsible for your hair loss?"

"No, not directly, at least," Samantha answered, fiddling with the gold band on her long fingers. "I did some research. It seems there is usually a genetic component involved. My dad had had a couple of bouts with alopecia areata—the bald spots—when he had a heart attack when I just a kid. When he finally came home from the hospital, I was afraid he was going to die. I was scared and worried. My hair fell out in the same kind of spots as he had. I've had a bald patch or two a few other times when I was under stress, but they were never a big deal and the hair always grew back. I learned from my research that stress, whether physical trauma or emotional trauma, is thought to be a trigger for alopecia. But the bottom line is, nobody really knows what causes alopecia and that's why NAAFs research is so vital.

"Eventually enough stress polluted my work environment to qualify it as a toxic dump. No matter what I did or didn't do, I couldn't please my boss. When I discovered I couldn't wear a wig because of a reaction to the backing that resulted in chronic yeast infections, things got really bad. Although the CEO of the company had no problem with my wearing hats, or even going without anything on my head, my own boss had a big problem with it. When I started wearing funky earrings I designed myself from brightly colored beads and unusual stones, and no make-up and only a shine on my bald head, he started looking for ways to get rid of me."

"How do you know that?" Desirae asked, her brows furrowing as she searched Samantha's face.

"Word gets around in an office with an active grapevine, and I

130

had a lot of friends." Samantha said. "Everything became obvious the day I went into his office and told him I didn't feel comfortable anymore and thought he wanted me to quit my job. He looked delighted and agreed just a little too quickly for his reaction to be anything but premeditated. He said he thought that would be best and bluntly told me that not only was I fat, which he found personally disgusting, but now I was bald and that didn't fit the image he wanted his office to portray. He wanted me to resign—after I finished the work he needed done for his project. Oh yeah, and I shouldn't go through Human Resources, I should just hand him my resignation when the work was completed.

Desirae's eyes widened like the eyes of a mongoose hot on the trail of a cobra. "Samantha, you're kidding, right?"

"I wish," Samantha replied. "Mostly I was stunned. I weighed about twenty pounds less than I had when he gave me that glowing ninety day evaluation. I understood that baldness altered my appearance greatly, but it didn't affect my ability to do the job."

"What did you tell him?"

"I said I needed a few days to think about it.

"And?"

"And he agreed to that."

"What did you do then?"

"I went home and talked to my husband about it and cried out my hurt and frustration. It was hard enough to lose my hair, but then to have somebody insinuate that I was ugly on top of ugly, well, that pretty much did me in. My husband was so incensed he was ready to help my boss to an early meeting with his Maker. Calming him down took all the energy I had left."

"Did you quit?"

"I felt defeated enough to. My husband told me to. But, the

more I thought about it the angrier I became. A few days later I went to the CEO and told him what happened."

"Good for you! What did he say?"

"He didn't say anything at first. His eyes went wide and his mouth dropped open. Then he said, 'If what you are saying is true, your boss was certainly in the wrong. In fairness, I'll need to hear his side of this issue too. I'll get back to you.'"

"My God, Samantha," Desirae said, waving her arm smack into the window next to her, "you should have sued them!" She put down her drink to rub her smarting hand.

"Funny you should say that. I thought about it, but what good would it have done?"

"Samantha, I am an employment attorney. You had grounds to sue, do you know that? And you would have won."

"Yeah, I figured as much. But I wouldn't have won because I was discriminated against for being bald. I would have won because he called me fat. It turns out baldness is not covered under the Americans with Disabilities Act. Baldness is not only acceptable for men, it is considered sexy—so why would there need to be any protection under the law for baldness? Bald women, however, don't share the same elevated status. I'm certain that had I walked into that initial interview bald, I never would have been hired. Since he expressed such virulent prejudice against fat people, I don't understand why he even hired me to begin with."

"What a bigot," Desirae hissed. "What finally happened?"

"Well," Samantha said, "it was all pretty anticlimactic. When the CEO questioned him, the guy owned what he'd said, brownie points for that, and I chose to quit working for him. Now I am very involved in raising alopecia awareness."

"That's just shit, just plain shit," Desirae said. "Something needs to be done to protect bald women from this kind of discrimination. Nobody should have to wear a wig if they choose not to, for whatever the reason! Men aren't expected to do that. Why should women?"

"From your mouth to God's ear," Samantha said, thoughtfully draining the last of the whiskey from her glass. "Yeah, Desirae, something should be done. I believe it will be in the years ahead. But for now, my bald head and sheer stubbornness in refusing to wear a head covering, despite pressure from my boss, and those bald heads of the brave women out there who share my beliefs and stand up for themselves, are bringing attention to alopecia and the crap many bald women have to deal with every day.

"Those of us who choose to push for the acceptance of female and child baldness use our own shiny heads to teach people about alopecia and its effects on women. At this point I can only be grateful for that pitiful man whose narrow minded prejudices brought me to a place of peace and purpose. Bad things can be used for good. Some of the most beautiful flowers grow out of the deepest piles of shit."

∂∘◌

So, there is Samantha's story. From California to the east coast, from the north to the south, her story reflects the workplace experiences of many bald women in the United States and around the world. Samantha's experience is indicative of the bigoted prejudice bald women face every day and must join forces to end, so that Alopecian children of both genders will be accepted to receive equal treatment in school and in the work place. As the children are our future, so our courage to embrace female baldness and educate those around us is their best hope to be defined for their character and what they do with their lives, rather than for the hair that is not on their heads.

Chapter 15

Flowers

Yesterday, when I finished writing the composite story of what happened to Samantha and the many others represented by her story, I turned off the computer and left the keyboard. I walked away feeling angry, frustrated and sad. In my Pollyanna heart, I cannot imagine anyone anywhere being treated so poorly because of their physical appearance. But, in the real world, as many have learned first-hand, it happens all the time.

What leaves me feeling grateful for having alopecia is the knowledge that I am not helpless to facilitate change. None of us are. Oh, we might not be in the place in time or circumstances to make change on a world-wide level, or even a national or state level. Still, every Alopecian is capable of positively impacting their immediate environment. Every Alopecian can bloom where they are potted. Every Alopecian can do what they can, where they are, with what they have. And every Alopecian can grow courage that flowers into actions.

BOLDLY BALD WOMEN

Discrimination can go on for years and years and years with no one doing anything to change it. Not the victims. Not the persecutors. Not the humanitarians. Then, so gradually that folks don't even sense the shift, one more person sees or hears of one more despicable incident and shares it with someone else. At some point people of the same mind find each other, and the balance tips. When enough people come together, what was once an unseen wound on the face of society is under a public spotlight, its septic corruption scrutinized for all to see.

I believe the reality for bald women and bald children is on the verge of a big change. What has not been spoken aloud is discussed more openly. What has been covered up is being bared. Alopecians are finding each other. The belief that bald is neither shameful nor ugly is growing. Bald women are finding their courage and beginning to take the actions that will change their status from hidden shadows in society to proud women who demand the same consideration as anyone with hair would have. The change is coming. Whether it comes quickly or slowly depends on how many Alopecians stand together and demand acceptance.

As there are people in the world who think it is okay to discriminate against others because of their gender, the color of their skin, or their sexual identity, there, too, are people who think it is acceptable to discriminate against female baldness. There are also many people out there who are perfectly comfortable to make room for bald women. But how will we find them if we keep our baldness hidden? How will we make employers see that what is in our heads does not equate to what is on our heads, if we don't first find our own courage to walk comfortably with the bald heads we want others to accept?

Here are some stories of women who have chosen to bloom where they are potted. Not all of their stories are as extreme as Sa-

135

BOLDLY BALD WOMEN

mantha's. The women and stories may be as different as chalk from cheese, but their emotional hurdles require the same strength and determination to vault. I celebrate their spirit. I admire their persistence. They are flowers in the Garden of Bald whose courage has come to fruition. Through the willingness of these amazing women to share, their courage will disperse as winged seeds on a wafting breeze, settle into the hearts of others facing alopecia and grow into yet more courage, self-confidence, and the determination to facilitate real change. May their stories provide you with interesting reading and inspiration.

❧

PAVING THE PATH
By Carol N. Jones,
Guelph, Ontario, Canada

SCHOOL

Although I've had alopecia since I learned to walk, it didn't affect my life until I attended school in Brampton, Ontario, where I was born and raised. I had alopecia areata until I was thirteen years old and my adoptive father treated me like I was any other "normal" kid. My mother, on the other hand, was embarrassed by my hair loss and persisted in rubbing a smelly topical ointment on my patches every night in desperation to cure me. When that wasn't working too effectively, over the course of a few years, I began wearing a shower cap over the solution applied to my head because heat and moisture apparently made a good breeding ground for hair follicles. I felt like a tropical houseplant!

As the balding worsened my adopted mother insisted on seeing a well-known dermatologist who did no better at curing me. That's when we saw a man in Montreal, Quebec, who I affection-

BOLDLY BALD WOMEN

*ately refer to as the witch doctor. He swung a pendulum over my
hand and did some palmistry, he mentioned that my nails looked
weak then sent us home with Rogaine.*

*By the time I started applying the Rogaine I was thirteen
and had alopecia totalis. I also began wearing a wig and when
I went to grade nine I ceased treatments altogether. During the
course of that time I was normally accepted by other children in
my neighborhood. I was a tomboy for the most part, however had
a few girls to play with during those feminine moments. I was the
only one of my local buddies to attend a special French Catho-
lic school, but there was one girl who lived on my street who also
went. I didn't like her very much, though, as my mother always
praised this girl on her beauty and intelligence. As I started wearing wigs, she had started modeling. It was almost like living up
to an older, over-achieving sibling and knowing that you'll never
measure up because it's just not you.*

*It wasn't my choice to lose my hair, nor was there anything
I could do about it. At school I was teased and taunted and if I
managed to make a friend, they weren't around for long. Anybody
willing to be the friend of a bald had their reputations tarnished.
I got into fights and, although I was never the one to instigate, I'd
be the one who ended it—or at least that was the goal. Somehow
these mishaps always turned out to be my fault, and I still believe
it was because the school took the same attitude as my mother.
Through nature's own natural selection the healthier looking kids,
kids that lied, were preferred over the sickly looking runt of the lit-
ter. I cried alone in my bedroom quite a bit throughout my school
years. Sometimes I'd vent to my father but it didn't do me any
good, he didn't get it. Nobody quite got it.*

I wanted to be a musician when I grew up and I became

more involved with music in high school. High school wasn't quite what I had expected or hoped. Unfortunately, I couldn't start over socially because too many kids from my elementary school came to the same high school and spread the news within our first week there. My first semester was horrible and I actually failed three classes that year. However, because I joined the school choir, I had the opportunity to be among many of the older students who were completely cool with my problem. Apparently, there were twin girls with alopecia at the school who had graduated the previous year. Somehow they managed to create a positive environment towards alopecia and this enabled me feel more comfortable. The music room became my home during my earlier high school days.

INTIMATE RELATIONS

My first boyfriend could not accept my baldness at all, and although we had a child together, our relationship did not last. My second boyfriend could accept that I was bald, he just didn't want to see it! For the first couple of years I wore my wig constantly, even to bed. I eventually managed to talk him into letting me wear a bandana to bed and shortly after that, I lost patience and ditched the wig. There was a lot of consideration that went into my decision to ditch the wig. When I had moved to Guelph, Ontario, we finally got the internet and I discovered alopecia groups on Yahoo and MSN. I had never really met anyone else with alopecia (except a high school friend's mom who avoided talking about it), and it was inspiring to see pictures of all these happy, bald Alopecians who led normal lives. Socially, this was difficult for my mate as he never had to deal with rude stares and comments. However, it slowly became easier for both of us.

BOLDLY BALD WOMEN

COMING OUT

Until this time, in 2001, my mother had always bought my expensive wigs. However, once on my own, I couldn't afford to get a new wig. The choice to go bald, I suppose, was made for me due to finances. Still, the fear of facing the world as a bald woman was something I had to let go of, come to terms with, and accept. I received much praise from my online communities and am grateful they were there for me, so to speak, to aide in my growth. I am still in contact with a few of these people a decade later and got the opportunity to meet some of them. Meeting other Alopecians is something I've been doing more, lately, since I decided I have grown and become strong enough to lead a support group. I was also lucky enough to have lunch with a group of ladies in Toronto and experienced seeing bald women like me for the first time.

It did take a few years to achieve my current comfort level. I began slowly going out bald in my backyard where only a few neighbors might see, then to the mall where I had to deal with my new image when I got questioned or stared at.

WORK PREJUDICE

My biggest challenge these days is keeping a smile on my face or my sense of humor when people stare rudely or ask silly questions. There's a big difference between an inquisitive look and one of either pity or disgust. I was furious at the news of an Owen Sound woman, who shaved her head for cancer and was asked to take the summer off with her kids so her hair could grow back. The restaurant owner described her appearance as appalling.

Even dread locks were a source of dread (pun intended) to

139

a woman who was hired (with dread locks) then fired for not adhering to the dress code. One thing I've learned through the years is that society will naturally push away anyone who doesn't fit into society's norm. I was being held back because of my appearance and although it was acceptable in the company policy for associates to wear a baseball hat with a company logo on it, I was somehow an exception to that rule.

Since the beginning of a new website called alopeciaworld. com, I have enjoyed a few great opportunities and continue to be an inspiration to Alopecians all over the world. I have written for another book and a Dutch magazine about alopecia. My support group has just celebrated its one year anniversary and the Children's Alopecia Project (CAP) asked me to be guest speaker at their conference. I did a music workshop with the kids, teaching them how to express themselves when no one around them gets it.

The thing that inspires me the most now is hearing about the kids with alopecia sharing their condition with not just their class but their entire school. This really seems to help them and is something I wish I could have done had it been acceptable at the time. There are so many young people with alopecia who have amazing attitudes!

Second to that, I am always happy to see another bald lady come to terms with her condition and go au naturel as someone once put it. My only fear or disappointment is that, even though it's gotten better over the years, alopecia is relatively unknown to the masses. Insurance coverage for those who want wigs is still relatively difficult to find.

We still have a long way to go before people stop assuming we're chemotherapy patients or understand that bald can be at-

*tractive too. That is why I will always do everything possible to put
us on the fast track to awareness and acceptance.*

—Carol

๛

From across the pond, Gwennan shares her journey to self-acceptance through her answers to my questionnaire.

YOUR ALOPECIA

Did you first experience alopecia as a child or as an adult?

I was twenty-five when the first patch appeared. I was getting my hair cut before my brother's wedding (May 2002,) when the hairdresser noticed a patch the size of a small coin. She suggested I pop along to my doctor to get it checked out.

**What type of alopecia do you have—areata, totalis, universalis?
Did you start out with one kind and end up with another?**

It began as areata (patches) progressing very quickly to totalis. Within six months I had lost everything (universalis). I was really upset when my eyelashes and eyebrows fell out. I felt so unattractive. I think eyelashes and eyebrows give shape and definition to your face. I felt so un-feminine. Looking at my twin sister's beautiful hair, eyelashes, and eyebrows made it all the more difficult for me to cope.

How long have you been dealing with alopecia?

It's been a little over seven years.

**Did something happen to trigger your hair loss, stress, illness, a
traumatic event?**

I had a number of stress factors at the time. Moving house, splitting up from a long-term relationship, and I was being bul-

141

lied at work. I also suffer with eczema, asthma and hay fever, and it has been suggested that they might be linked to alopecia.

Does anyone else have alopecia in your family?

No.

Did you seek medical treatment? What was done and what effect did it have?

I did seek medical advice. My GP prescribed an anti-fungal cream, having only inspected my scalp from two feet away. I was working with a pharmacist at the time, so I asked her advice. She said that it was definitely not fungal and to go back to the GP. The GP just told me that it was nothing to worry about and sent me away. My sister and I researched on the internet, and were more and more convinced that it was alopecia.

YOUR REACTIONS

What were your initial reactions to hair loss?

Devastation. I was traumatized. Of course the more I worried, the worse it became. I have a twin sister, and I am ashamed to say that I felt bitter that this was happening to me. Losing my hair on top of severe eczema and asthma, I felt unable to cope. I became very low and all my confidence was knocked out of me.

What did you do to process what was happening and move forward?

I had a lot of support from friends and family, so I was lucky. I have always had a fighting spirit, having coped with the eczema and asthma all my life. So eventually, I just tried to get on with my life. My sister, in particular, was a rock to me.

What made you decide not to wear a wig if you don't?

To begin, I actually wore bandanas. I felt this was a funky way to cope with having no hair. I was adamant that I would

142

never wear a wig. Though, four years later, I was persuaded to give them a go. For the best part of two to two and a half years it was fabulous. I felt more feminine and confident. I loved the feeling of having hair again. Though given that my second wig fell apart as did the third and fourth, it was a very stressful time. The wig company actually blamed me for the way I must have cared for it.

To be treated this way has caused me a lot more stress, to the point of taking anti-depressants. It brought back similar feelings to that of losing my hair all those years ago. It made me re-evaluate why I was wearing wigs, and why I had not just gone bald to begin with. Surely, wearing a wig is designed to make your life less stressful. I can honestly say that I wish I had never considered wigs in the first place. At least, I gave them a go.

What prompted you to explore letting go of wigs/head coverings?

Having been through so many expensive wigs (in the region of £6,000 GBP) that have fallen apart, and having been blamed for this, I became very depressed and felt as though I was trapped. I felt the choice of wearing wigs had been taken away from me, even though I had been considering the option of going without for some time. The final blow came when wig number four ripped in half. I went on a week's girls' holiday to Cyprus, where I plucked up the courage to go without anything on my head. I decided that now was the time to go bald, especially just a few days away from International Alopecia Day™.

The first day back at work after my holiday was very nerve-wracking, and even though most people knew I had alopecia, revealing my bald head had been something very personal to me over the last seven years. The first time I went bald to work, I felt a huge sense of empowerment. Colleagues, friends and family have all been fantastic, and have given me the confidence I needed to go for it every day.

Did anything happen that made you laugh?

My friends, family, and I try to make light of my alopecia. Not to make a joke about it, but to take it at face value and turn the negatives into positives.

My boyfriend used to put my old wig on, which always made me laugh! My nephew likes to slap (gently, might I add) my bald head, which makes him and me crease with laughter. I joke that one day I'm going to walk into a hair salon and ask for a perm! I work for a team that helps support doctors who struggle with behavioural, language and communication problems. One doctor came for an appointment after I had ditched my wig and blurted out, "What's happened to you?"

Although he was abrupt, I couldn't help laughing, thinking this is the reason you are here. Another Korean doctor asked me whether I had gotten a new hairstyle!

Did anything happen that left you feeling self-conscious or sad or embarrassed?

Unexpected visitors when I was bald at home (before the bald days). I would get annoyed with friends, who would invite people over at a time when I was not comfortable with people I didn't know seeing me bald. A constant worry. But I have to say, that feeling has disappeared since taking the plunge to go boldly bald!

Comments made by people who don't understand alopecia have hurt, but I try to remember that it's only because they have probably never heard of alopecia.

I used to feel very bitter when a group of my girlfriends and I would get ready for a night out. They would be doing their hair and I would feel left out, angry, bitter and jealous. Nowadays, I have an extra fifteen minutes in bed in the morning not having to wash, dry or style my hair. I save money on hair products. Swimming is a lot easier when not having to deal with taking off a wig and putting it back on. Plus, on holiday, you get a lovely brown head and keep a lot cooler!

What is your greatest fear about alopecia?

It used to be the thought of never having hair again. That people wouldn't love me for who I was. Fear that I had to cope with alopecia for the rest of my life. The constant explanation of it to new friends/colleagues. I feel a strong sense of relief now that I am bald. I no longer have a burden to carry around, worrying whether or not my wig will fall apart, or if people can tell I'm bald underneath this bandana.

Now? I am bald. And people can see this straight away. Of course, the majority of people will think chemotherapy and the minority might consider alopecia. As long as I am confident and happy in myself, it is obvious to see that I am a happy and healthy individual who happens to have no hair, who is fortunate not to have to go through chemotherapy, and a person who smiles a hell of a lot.

What is your greatest hope about alopecia?

That women who lose their hair get offered support and advice. Counseling has helped me come to terms with my alopecia and given me the confidence to go for it with my baldness. It is a long journey, I can't deny that. But as long as women are given the best possible support, half the battle is already won. I was never offered any counseling, and the support groups that I did go to were more aimed at a group of middle-aged women meeting for a pub crawl. It was a farce.

BOLDLY BALD WOMEN

Have you come to a place of acceptance over hair loss? If so, how did you get there? If not, how are you feeling currently?

I have been in counseling for almost twelve months. This has been an incredible help to me. Friends and family can offer unconditional support, which is, of course, equally important, but seeing a counselor, who is completely impartial and will listen and suggest ways of coping, has changed the way I think about my alopecia. I now know that with or without hair, I am still Gwen. It has been a tough and sometimes frightening experience. But it also has given me the confidence to be who I am. It has helped me get over my fear of what others think.

Slowly, I began accepting myself by telling colleagues at work about my alopecia. I would also tell new people I met. This gave me a confidence boost and made me realize that it really didn't matter that I had no hair. Gradually, I went from explaining my hair loss to going completely bald—something I never thought I would be able to do.

There is a lady I've seen who walks around Cardiff (who I have tried tracking down) who is also bald. Even though we have never met, her courage gave me the guts to go for it. I felt as though I was not alone.

How has alopecia changed the way you think others view you?

It has taught me to be less superficial and to take people for who they are. It has also taught me a lot about other people. Those who make the snide remarks are not worth knowing or even explaining to. I would like to be treated the way I treat others. I realize now that alopecia is just one very, very small part of me. My character as a person is who I am, not some long blonde hair.

How has coping with alopecia changed the way you see yourself?

It's hard to sometimes remember that I need to give myself

more credit, as I am often told. I try to see myself as a confident and strong woman who has had battles most of her life, but can still hold down a really good job, who has a beautiful home, a fantastic family, a wonderful boyfriend and bunch of friends. I have got to where I am because of who I am. I try to remind myself that a lot of people would have given up and hidden away. Having a fighting and uncompromising spirit, I have never wanted to let anything or anyone hold me back. This spirit was trodden upon but somehow, with the support of a lot of people around me, has shone through.

YOUR FAMILY
How did your family react to your hair loss (parents, siblings, spouse, children, and extended relatives)?

I have a twin sister. It was very hard for her to see me go through hair loss. However, she was a huge barrel of strength. My parents were also fantastic. They all rallied round to offer support.

Was it easy to talk about your alopecia and your feelings about it?

Not particularly. I became quite low and withdrawn and felt there was little point in talking to anyone, as I was told by the dermatologist that it was too late to do anything. In a way, I got fed up of talking about it.

If your family was supportive, how did they show that support?

Just by being there. I was living with my sister at the time, so we spent a lot of time together. I couldn't have coped without her. My parents lived an hour's drive away, but I saw them regularly. My sister would leave cheery little notes for me, which always made me smile. Mum often came across to Cardiff and we would just spend time together, which always helped.

147

BOLDLY BALD WOMEN

Did your hair loss impact your intimate relations with spouse/significant other? If so, how?

    My relationship was with a guy before my alopecia developed. I hadn't had a boyfriend in all that time. Any guy I did meet was put off by my hair loss. Some were okay about it, but I never found anyone who loved me for who I was, until recently. I have met the most amazing and wonderful guy. He actually prefers me bald and he loves me for me. He's been a real pillar of strength and has also given me the courage and confidence to go bald, because he thinks I'm beautiful without hair.

Did your family's reaction make it easier or more difficult for you to cope?

    Without them, I would not have coped.

Was there anyone person in your life who made coping with alopecia easier? What did they do or not do that was most helpful to you?

    My twin sister, Mum and Dad. We have always been a close family. Sometimes I feel as though I am a burden: the daughter with the never-ending problems. But they have always, no matter what, been there for me. Mum has always been this amazing person who has basically taught me that we can get through any situation, no matter how difficult. She had a very hard time when I was born, because I developed severe eczema. I had to be bathed, creamed and bandaged daily. With two other siblings to care for, this made life very tough indeed. So, over the years, Mum has been almost part of me. She is the one who has given me that fighting spirit. Without her, I'm not sure I would have coped with my eczema and certainly not my alopecia.

What was said or done that was insensitive or hurtful?

    At the wedding of one of my best friends, I was seated at

a table and about to have the wedding breakfast when another guest, who I had never met, approached the table. At the time I was in my bandana stage. I wore a beautiful black dress with bright pink flowers attached to the front. My Mum had made me a matching bandana, which I thought was quite striking. The guest proceeded to say, "I didn't realize we had a nun as a guest."

What did you most want to hear from your family?

There is really nothing anyone CAN say. They couldn't have said that my hair would grow back, because no one can say that. I guess the best help is if your family can be honest with you. Self-image is crucial at this time. You are so utterly self-conscious, that you want an honest opinion.

THE WORLD IN GENERAL
Did your friendships change in any way?

No. My true friendships only became stronger.

Were there any negative impacts on your job when you went to work without head coverings? Were you told or 'encouraged' to cover your baldness at work, or were you threatened or fired?

Absolutely not. My work colleagues have been extremely encouraging and helped me believe that I could do it.

Was there somewhere you felt very accepted? What did others do to encourage you that helped?

Amongst friends and family for sure. Though most of what you feel is in your head, a majority of people would only think positively, so I am now informed!

What did others do that grated on your last nerve?

Assume that I am going through chemo.

BOLDLY BALD WOMEN

Did you get confused for a chemo therapy patient? What did you do or say to correct the false perception?

All the time. I explained that I was lucky to be healthy, that it is only alopecia and that I am far happier bald than wearing wigs or bandanas. What are the most tactless things people have ever asked/said? I think just making assumptions. I guess this boiled down to education. Most people are ignorant about alopecia, and it is up to us to teach people. The guy at the wedding really upset me.

What are the kindest, most thoughtful things people have ever said/done?

That I am more beautiful bald.

What would you like people to know about asking the obvious questions about why you are bald?

That I am still a human being, like everyone else. To accept that people are different and not to make generalized assumptions. Taking a tactful approach always helps!

What would you most like me to know about you and your story?

It happened to me seven years ago. It has been a long and tough journey, but I am certainly at a turning point, because I have had the courage to go bald. I am Gwennan, with or without hair. It is what is inside that matters. I am very lucky to have a fantastic family, a great group of friends and an amazing boyfriend, who all see me for who I am. I just wish I had known more about this seven years ago and had explored my options through counseling. I think that GPs need to be more aware of alopecia, offering counseling as standard treatment.

—Gwennan

BOLDLY BALD WOMEN

⤔⤕

Sarah, who began her story in You're Not Alone, continues here:

My first experience with alopecia took place when I was thirteen. Alopecia impacted me deeply. It changed the way I looked at the world and the way I saw myself. Prior to my hair falling out I was a fairly attractive, popular young teen. I was, like so many others my of age, very caught up in superficial appearances. When my hair fell out I was suddenly thrust into a new awareness. This awareness did not come easily. It was very painful. I had always been a fairly sensitive and somewhat introverted person, and losing my hair to alopecia caused me to go further inward.

I have gone through different phases during these few years with alopecia in which I tried out different ways of being with my hair loss. After the first few months of losing hair, I came to the decision one day that I no longer wanted to watch, day after day, as each new pile of hair greeted me in the morning. It was then that I got some hair clippers and shaved my head. This was an empowering choice and act, amidst an experience in which I felt I had absolutely no control. Up until this time I had worn hats to conceal my alopecia. My total baldness was new and although it was scary and uncomfortable I went through my daily life completely bald for over a year. It was during this time that I experienced many of the negative reactions from others. I often felt afraid of going out in public and avoided social situations a great deal of the time.

After about a year and half, my hair began to re-grow and for a few months it appeared as though my bout with alopecia was ending. However, this was not the case and once again the bald patches reappeared. This second time around was almost harder in some ways because I had experienced a reprieve and hoped that it was over, only to be struck again. I fell into a very deep depression. For some time I even considered suicide.

It was truly a dark chapter in my life. I look back on it now and it feels like another lifetime, so far away. However, I know that those experiences are still with me and have helped to shape the woman I am today.

I decided to try out wigs. Unfortunately the first wig I got was not a very good one and it was spotted by kids a mile away. I was teased mercilessly because of it. I did at one point have a human hair wig that was quite similar to my own hair. I wore it for a period of time and somewhat enjoyed the feeling of not standing out, and of not being the brunt of negative attention. However, I never really got accustomed to wearing a wig all the time.

At some point in time, approximately three years after the patches appeared, my hair began to re-grow although none of the treatment options had helped. My hair grew back seemingly of its own accord and I had normal hair growth for approximately eight years after that.

My second experience with alopecia began in my mid-twenties. Ever since I was a teen I had had hormonal disturbances, which manifested in many ways including irregular periods, ovarian cysts, anxiety and depression. In my mid-twenties I was still experiencing these issues and my hair began thinning on the top/front of my head. This type of alopecia was different than the alopecia I had experienced as a teen and part of me wondered if I was imagining it, because I definitely had a fear of my hair falling out again. I began finding hair in the shower again and counting how many strands fell out every day. Disturbingly, it was well over the average. Again I went to a number of doctors. I tried Rogaine and spironolactone. I went on birth control pills. I tried natural alternatives, many different hair growth products. Still, my hair continued to fall out. This went on over a period of about five years until I could no longer hide the issue. My hair was so thin on top that it was virtually invisible.

Finally, at the age of twenty-nine, I was diagnosed with an endocrine disorder. This disorder causes major disruptions in my hormonal system, which has caused me to manifest this particular form of alopecia, known as androgenetic alopecia. It is the same type of alopecia that causes male pattern baldness. This has been somewhat difficult for me to tolerate as well. As a woman I find there is something discomforting about having male pattern baldness. However, as with all aspects of this condition, I have come to terms with the fact that my body is unique and it just is what it is.

However, with that said, this time around I still struggled deeply with my hair loss. I felt ugly, unattractive. I wondered what was wrong with me. Why did I have this problem? Had I done something to cause it? Could it be reversed like the last time? After many years of trying different drugs and different therapies I finally came to the conclusion that, for my own sanity, I needed to let it go. I needed to stop trying to make my hair grow. I needed to find a place of acceptance.

When I got to this point, I felt relieved. Once again I found myself shaving my head, deciding that doing so felt better than living with the alternative of my hair continuing to slowly fall out. I decided I would try out some wigs again. After all, the wigs nowadays are much better than they were twenty years ago. I've accumulated several wigs since then. I have some human hair wigs, the vacuum type, and some synthetic wigs, in many different

153

colors and styles. There have been times when I wear them quite often, and times when I don't wear a single one for over a year or more.

Over the past year or so, I have mainly worn beautiful head scarves in public. I wrote a blog entry about this on Alopecia World, which explains this decision:

For the past year or so I have not worn a wig. Instead I have mainly chosen to wear head scarves in public. I have also gone completely bald. Over the years I have gone through a continuous inner struggle with this issue, whether to just go bald, wear a wig, or a head-covering. I wonder how many others face this same issue and/or feel similarly about it. Sometimes I enjoy wearing a wig. Playing with different looks can be fun and there are times, especially when doing something formal, that it feels good to have hair. However, on some level, I also find that, for me, wearing a wig is pretty stressful. I expend precious energy wondering how it looks to others and whether people can tell that it's a wig.

Then there's also the issue of feeling somehow false in a wig. The feeling of being false is one of the most fascinating aspects of the experience to me, because I know it is entirely my own perception that creates this feeling. Other people who don't know me, and never get to know me well, don't know the difference anyway. Those who do know me know that I am the same person with or without a wig. So, why the sense of deception? I think there are many reasons, and I'm not sure I have a handle on all of them yet. One is that people make a lot of judgments about others based on their appearances. People interact differently with me, for instance, depending on whether I am wearing a short, brunette wig or a longish blonde wig. In some way, when I am meeting new people in a wig, I always feel like the wig somehow colors my inter-

action with the other person.

On the other hand, when I have gone completely bald, I have encountered an entire spectrum of responses from people, ranging from sympathy from those who assume I am fighting cancer, to embarrassment on the part of others, to rudeness and downright hostile energy. So, in that sense, not wearing a wig certainly does not spare me from the mis-perceptions or judgment of others.

I find being a bald woman in an appearance-oriented, materialistic culture a really interesting study in human behavior—my own and other people's. I no longer struggle internally over my hair loss and have come to accept it. Personally, I think my bald head is rather beautiful. If I lived in a cabin in the woods with people close to me I'd go bald all the time. So, why the choice to cover up? For one thing, I am a very sensitive and intuitive person. I can feel other people's energies and sense judgment a mile away. Although I know I don't need to take any of that on, it can get pretty exhausting being bombarded all the time by the curious, misguidedly sympathetic and/or aggressive glances, stares, words etc. Being an openly bald woman is sort of like wearing a target. You draw attention to yourself whether you want it or not.

I think, within our culture, there is also a fear of bald women—women who do not allow themselves to be constrained by society's measure of beauty—are a threat to the status quo. I think women who intentionally shave their heads, without having any type of an alopecia issue, are making a very powerful and intentional statement about these misogynistic beauty standards. More power to them. I'm also aware that sometimes others interpret my baldness within this context, assuming I am trying to make a statement by being bald. Perhaps in some sense I am, but truthfully, any statement I make with my appearance is more like a by-product of the awareness which has grown directly out of my experiences with alopecia.

So, that's kind of it in a nutshell. My experiences with alopecia have changed my life in many ways and helped shape my perspective. They have given me deeper insight into myself, and into what I value, both in myself, and in other people. I've learned that my beauty, like the beauty of so many others, goes much deeper than skin-deep. I'm also much more likely to make discernments regarding other people based on a true interaction with them rather than on the way they look. I think that's a healthier, more open way to be. I've had to learn a level of self-acceptance that I might not otherwise have achieved if I had not had alopecia. For many people, our sense of self-worth is very tied up in the way we look and whether or not we are found acceptable, or attractive, by other people. Letting all of that fall away, or, at least being able to sort it out and be responsible for my own sense of self-worth, has been a gift alopecia has given me.

Sure, there are times when I wish I had hair, but nowadays those times are few and far between. I don't choose to spend my energy wishing circumstances beyond my control could be different than they are. Life is happening now. This is who I am and I'm going to make the best of it.

—Sarah

❧

Megan Adair from Norfolk, Virginia shares her process to accept her baldness.

It was a Tuesday. I was fifteen years old, and like every Tuesday, I would go to the doctor, receive my treatment, and then go home. On that particular Tuesday, however, something different occurred. I didn't follow my normal routine. It was a strange day for me. I had the routine memorized like the back of my hand, but that Tuesday was the day it all changed.

I sat in the waiting room of the doctor's office. I had always hated the plain gray walls that began to blur when you stared at them for a long time. I hated the faint whisper of the ticking clock that held a meaningless melody. I hated it all. I laid my head back against the gray, and gently I closed my eyes. I thought back to that first day when I entered the office. I remembered it like a bad dream one longs to escape. I was ten years old. I lived a simple life until I entered that prison. Up until then my life was carefree, uncomplicated and filled with laughter. Little did I know that something was happening to me that would change the course of my life forever.

"Mom, what's wrong with me?" I asked.

"Nothing sweetheart, you're perfect. We're just here to find out what's going on." She gave me that loving smile that always comforted me. I sat there waiting anxiously for the doctor to call me back to the examining room.

This is a strange place, I thought to myself. I didn't like the way it reeked of old people and bad candles. It was cold like a frigid ice box. I hated it, and it was only my first time.

"Megan Adair," called a nurse from behind the door. She was a short lady with short gray hair. She fit right in with all the other senior citizens. I approached her and walked through the door. I was beginning to get nervous. I was shaking and my heart began to race. I could hear it like the rhythm of a drum.

"Dr. Poinsette will be with you in a few moments," the nurse said in a quiet voice.

Again, I waited. I was so curious to finally figure out what was happening to me. I couldn't understand why my hair was falling out. Why was this happening to me? I couldn't remember if I had made mistakes for which I hadn't been forgiven. Did I deserve this?

"Hi there Megan, I'm Doctor Poinsette." She was a middle-aged woman. She had midnight black hair, with a few gray ones mixed in. She had a friendly face, and I instantly began to warm up to her.

"What are you here for?" she asked.

I explained that my hair was falling out in the shower and when I brushed it. I told her I had noticed that strands of my hair were everywhere. She asked me a series of questions, which were all followed by the answer, "No." She asked me if she could take a look at my head, and I willingly agreed. As she ran her fingers through my straight, honey kissed, brown hair, I felt her fingers run across bare scalp. I knew it had come to this, I just knew it. A tear cautiously slid down my cheek. She lifted my head and looked at me.

She let out a sigh, and spoke, "Megan, I am so sorry to tell you this, but you have a spot on your head with no hair."

No hair, no hair, no hair. That phrase repeated itself like a broken record in my mind. I began to weep.

She told me, "You have alopecia areata. Alopecia areata is a type of hair loss that occurs when your immune system mistakenly attacks hair follicles, which is where hair growth begins. The damage to the follicle is usually not permanent. Experts do not know why the immune system attacks the follicles. It cannot kill you, and there is no cure."

She told me everything that came along with this disease and how apparently I wasn't alone. A lot of people had it. She

BOLDLY BALD WOMEN

talked about the different forms of treatment. I began to tune out. My mind was running wild. I came back to earth when she asked me what I wanted to do about it. I didn't know what I wanted, or even what to say. The only thing I did know was that I wanted to get rid of it.

We chose a treatment where I would have shots of cortisone injected into my head where the hair was non-existent. She handed me a piece of paper and said, "I'll see you next week to start treatment." As I slowly trudged out of the building, I turned and looked back. There was no telling what my future would hold. I opened my eyes. The flashback was over and I was sitting in Dr. Poinsette's examining room. I wondered how I got there. When did I get up and start walking? I guess my mind was so focused on my past that I had no clue what I was doing.

Her room was so boring. It was one color, white. White desk, white walls, white bed, everything was white. I was always so cold sitting on that stiff medical bed. And every Tuesday I waited. But today was different for me. Today I was stopping my treatment for good. And the only thing I could think about was how my whole life had been altered by this condition. I closed my eyes once again. I couldn't see the faint picture of the memory of my life four years ago. Four whole years of my life had been erased. Like a drawing on a desk that eventually gets cleaned, my drawing had disappeared. Another flashback came.

As I crawled out of bed, I looked at myself in the mirror. "Today's the first day of high school," I said in a nonchalant tone. As I looked at my reflection, I saw big brown eyes the size of boulders. I saw cherry red lips and pale cheeks. But I also saw a girl with no hair. Yes, I had other features, but the only thing I could truly see was a monster. I was a freak. I placed the wig firmly on my head, brushed it to the tips, and stared. You could tell. I knew *you could tell it was a wig. Everyone was going to figure it out. So I grabbed my brown, worn down beanie and gently slid it over my wig. I was safe under my hat. It was like a baby blanket protecting a child. I was now ready to face the day and go to school.*

"Mom," I yelled as I walked downstairs.

"Yes, honey," she answered.

"Ma, what do you think they're gonna say?" I asked.

"They will probably be jealous that you are allowed to wear a hat and they're not," she replied.

"Yeah, I guess, but what if they all stare and make fun of me?"

"Then you can remember that I love you, and that you are beautiful," my mother said sincerely. I gave her a smile, and with a tear resting in the corner of my eye I headed to school.

As I approached the rusted doors of Daniel High School, I began to second guess my confidence, and I began to quiver. I couldn't do this! What was I thinking? I was scared to death for what awaited me inside. I stood outside for a moment, and where I found the courage to go inside, I will never know. When I walked in, I could feel every single eye in that building peering at me. It seemed they were waiting for me like an animal waiting to kill its prey. But honestly, I can't say I blamed them for that. To them, I was the new freshman, who mysteriously wore a hat to school. Truthfully, I was a fourteen-year-old girl who was hiding a big secret under a simple brown hat.

"Um, do you have permission to wear a hat in the building?" was the question I received most that day. All those teachers must have thought, "Wow, here's another hoodlum that we have to deal with." My replies were, "Yes ma'am, I do," or "Yes, sir, I do."

I went through most of the day being called names like hat girl, or people asking me "How is the Chemo going?" and when

160

was I planning on kicking the bucket. I tried to ignore their snickering, but it was so hard to escape from their evil comments. I left school that day torn to pieces.

When I got home, I lay down on my ivory carpet and cried. I did this for the next three months. Every day I cried. Crying soon became second nature to me. I often found myself begging my depression to please cut to the chase and end. I could be summed up by three words, depressed, hated, and miserable.

One day my mother said to me, "Enough of this, I can't bear to see you hurting yourself like this any longer."

I began to sob. "Mom," I said. "I'm ugly, I miss it, I miss being able to play sports and swim. I miss the wind through my hair. I can't even remember how it felt to have the wind through my hair. Why can't I look like everyone else? How come they all got lucky? Mom, I hate that school and I hate myself. I can't do this any longer. I just don't know how."

Silence was all I received. I knew my mother didn't even know what to say. No one could possibly know the right thing to say, because no one truly understood how I felt. So, she wrapped me up in her arms and cried with me.

I started a new treatment a few days later. It was an ointment that the doctor would put on my head every week. It was called DCPC. It was a clear, odorless liquid. It burned as if it were a toxic poison that was slowly taking someone's life. With one touch to my scalp my whole body would ache. It was like a mixture of poison ivy and sun burn. Painful, oh yes, it was hell. But at that point, I was prepared to try anything to make my hair grow back.

I visited the doctor once a week, every Tuesday for a year. Nothing happened. Not a single hair grew back on my head that year. I was quickly labeled, not only as a human experiment, because I had tried every single treatment there was, but also as a hopeless case, because none of those treatments worked. I was in-curable.

I finished my freshman year completely bald. As summer approached I was given a gift. In my eyes it was the most beautiful thing I had ever seen. Fifteen inches of real human hair and it was mine. It was long and dark and everything I had always dreamt of. When I slid the beautiful, silky wig onto my head I was trans-formed from a monster into something beautiful. I loved it, and for the first time in a long time I was actually happy.

And with that happiness, off came my hat. I didn't need it anymore, because I felt normal again. After that, it was hard to be envious of someone else. Now, other people were envious of me. They all wanted my hair. And it felt good to feel like I finally be-longed. It was like I had a new place in the world.

After summer, and my fifteenth birthday, I went back to school. I was confident. I had no hat, which brought no jokes, and no more malicious whispers. I was a normal high school kid. I did not have any hair, but I was content with my life. I looked beauti-ful, and my condition was almost a thing of the past. Yes, I still dealt with it every day, but I could actually look into the mirror and see that the person staring back at me was pretty and no one could take that away from me.

As I opened my eyes and adjusted them to the light, I real-ized I was back, back to the same old white room which had con-sumed my life for five years.

Knock, knock," said Dr. Poinsette as she entered the room. "How did you react to treatment last week?" she asked with hope-ful eyes.

"Nothing happened again, big surprise," I rolled my eyes. I was so sick of this let down every week. "I'm ..." It was hard to say what I was trying to get out. The words were stuck in my throat

like glue stuck on paper. "I'm stopping treatment." I hated giving up, I had fought for so long, but I knew this was what I had to do. She gave me a confused look. "Dr. Poinsette," I began with a soft voice, "I have been coming to you for five years and nothing has happened. It's not worth it anymore. I'm just gonna let it be and see what happens. But, I want to thank you for never giving up on me and trying to heal me." I began to cry. "I think it's time for me to heal myself," I said.

"You are the strongest person I know, Megan. I can't wait to see what you're meant to do for the world. You were given this condition for a reason, but you have handled this battle beautifully, and I look up to you. Come back and see me in a few months," said Dr. Poinsette.

"I will," I promised. When I walked out, I said goodbye to that office, and goodbye to the place that changed my life forever. And I said goodbye to someone who never lost hope in me, even though I saw none in myself. While I drove away, I thought quietly, now I just have to trust in Fate and trust in myself that I won't give up. If my hair comes back, that's great. If it never comes back, that's okay. I know that I don't need to have a full head of hair to be beautiful. I am a fifteen-year-old girl with no hair, and I know who I am. So, think about it, who are you?

When I look back, losing my hair was almost a blessing. Most people would probably say that I am crazy for stating that. It's true though, having no hair has taught me amazing things. It allows me to see qualities in people that others tend to overlook. If I have learned anything in the past five years, it's that you are not defined but how you look or by what you have. You are defined by who you are and what you do with yourself. Life is not given to us so we can spend it hiding behind our own insecurities. We are all fools for caring about what other people think. Trust me. I spent days and weeks worrying about what everyone thought of me. When all along I should have been paying attention to the person I was becoming, and I wish I could have seen all the people I was hurting by hating myself. Don't let something take over your life. Set yourself free from the opinions of others, and allow yourself to see people for who they truly are. For the record, I will probably never have a full head of hair ever again, but that doesn't matter. I am me. And I am free.

—Megan

❧⁓

COMMON THREADS

Different women, different countries, different stories, yet, despite fear, ridicule, job discrimination and emotional pain, they have found their way to very similar conclusions.

❧⁓

We still have a long way to go before people understand that bald can be attractive too. That is why I will always do everything possible to put us on the fast track to awareness and acceptance.

It has been a long and tough journey, but I am certainly at a turning point, because I have had the courage to go bald. I am Gwennan, with or without hair.

I don't choose to spend my energy wishing circumstances beyond my control could be different than they are. Life is happening now. This is who I am and I'm going to make the best of it.

If I have learned anything in the past five years, it's that you are not defined by how you look or by what you have. You are defined by who you are and what you do with yourself. For the record, I will probably never have a full head of hair ever again, but that doesn't matter. I am me. And I am free.

ॐ

Free. Free of insecurity. Free of anxiety from being discovered. Free of the opinions, fears, and prejudices of others. Free to leave the whole issue of baldness behind and move on with your life. Female baldness, regardless of cause, should be a non-issue. As more and more women walk together with strength and in one accord, the day will come when it will become just that—a non-issue. And on our way to that end, there are so many lessons to learn about ourselves, so many blessings to reap and hold in our hearts, so many other women and children to benefit from our courage and persistence in the face of difficulties.

As Megan put it so well, *"You are defined by who you are and what you do with yourself."*

Who are you? And what will you do with yourself and the blessing of life you have been given?

CHAPTER 16
RE: Joyce

꙾

Life isn't about finding yourself, it's about creating yourself.
—George Bernard Shaw

꙾

RE: JOYCE

Here is Joyce's take on living boldly bald. Reading Joyce's response to my questionnaire, I learned she is a jewelry designer and I had to laugh. Call it a God thing as I do, call it serendipity or whatever you choose, I had been looking for someone to help me develop an idea for jewelry for bald women (regardless of the cause of their hair loss) and those supporting them. Joyce and I have become fellow adventurers in this endeavor. We have had so much fun getting to know each other and designing jewelry for the website boldlybaldwomen.com. Here's Joyce's story.

My Life as a Bald Fashion Icon
Once upon a time I had hair. Then it was gone. Poof!

BOLDLY BALD WOMEN

AGE 12

At about twelve years old I developed alopecia areata. I was born with eczema so dermatologists were no strangers to me. I developed a bald spot on my head about the size of a quarter. Mom dragged me back to the handsome doctor on the fashionable east side of Providence, Rhode Island.

"Hmm. Alopecia." He sounded very matter of fact.

Didn't feel that way to me. Here I was already convinced that I was a freak with my eczema and now I was losing my hair. Great. Doctor put something on the spot that burned a bit. Then I sat under some magic light. Guess he decided that I was stressed too—so he gave me a prescription for Valium. Here I was, a blotchy, pre-pubescent child with bald spots. There was no discussion about the prognosis, long term outlook, or what this disease was all about. Take these pills and come back in a week or two weeks or a month. The more I thought about it, the more hair I lost. Now there were two spots, later three. Spot number one began filling in. Sometimes, I thought that if I could ignore it, the fall would stop. Eventually, it did. Doc chased those bald spots around my head for a few years, and then I had hair, more or less. I lived in constant fear that this would start again. Checked my comb and brush daily. Checked my head in the mirror. Like a good little patient I took my Valium every day—for years.

AGE 18

My buddy Al was back again. Not sure if it was after a romance break up or just the stress of being eighteen. I must say being eighteen in 1969 wasn't all bad. The world was in chaos, but the world of style and fashion was upside down. My wavy (naturally unruly) hair was actually in style. Enough with iron-

ing my hair or winding my hair around soup cans. It no longer mattered that I was not blond with big boobs. Surfer Girl had been replaced by Annie Hall. My new found freedom came crashing down when my hair started to fall out again. Just like before, one spot then more. I had figured out what Valium was a while back and stopped taking it. New doctor now gave me Atarax. Not sure what it was, but my mom said they gave it to some of the patients at the state mental hospital where she worked. Okay, I'll try it. After all it was 1969 and it might give me a buzz (instead of a buzz cut). Eventually the hair grew back.

24-ISH

Got married at twenty-one. Had a son, Jesse, at twenty-two. My beautiful child was (and still is) the light of my life. Got divorced at twenty-four—charges—mental cruelty. Unfortunately, my marriage evaporated pretty quickly. I remember being in court testifying about lots of things, but I remember how everybody gasped when I mentioned that my hair had been falling out as a result of the stress in my relationship. I had just cut my hair very short and I am sure they thought I had lost it all. Same story—lost some, lost more, grew back. By now, this was a familiar process, and hair was the least of my worries at this point in my life. I had a job and a wonderful child.

Many years with hair followed this. Surely, I must be cured. Maybe I had outgrown it. I continued to check for spots and count hairs in my comb and brush waiting for the hair loss to reappear. Years of looking over your shoulder can give you a big pain in the neck.

BOLDLY BALD WOMEN

52-ISH

In late spring/early summer of 2003, my son called me, very upset.

"Mom my hair is falling out!"

I can't believe I just said, "Oh well, you ARE a guy—my dad had male pattern baldness."

He said, "No—it is falling out all over my head in handfuls!"

He thought he was dying. I forgot that he was only two when I had my last bout with alopecia. He had no idea what was going on. I tried to reassure him. I told him about alopecia and that I had alopecia when I was younger, and that my hair grew back. I was devastated. I prayed to God to take my hair and leave him out of this deal. Well, it didn't work out quite that way.

Two weeks later, my hair started to fall out. It wasn't long before we were both completely bald. We worried about each other and thought little about what was happening to us individually. As it began falling out, I knew this time that it was all going. I got my hair cut and styled to cover the first areas balding and told my family, friends, and co-workers that I was losing my hair. Friends of mine, who have a boutique that sells wigs, helped me get some wigs to wear.

When I could no longer cover the spots, I started wearing wigs to work. Every day in my life was a costume party! I got more compliments on my wig hair than when I had my own. I decided to make the best of it, and I bought wigs in every color. I was platinum blonde one day and red the next. When people commented on my hair, I always explained that I was wearing a wig and told them about alopecia. Meanwhile, my son lost all of the hair on his head. I bought him twelve hats for Christmas that year. When

169

my hair became very sparse, I decided it was time to shave it off. I felt better after shaving my head. I thought that rather than looking sick, I just looked bald.

After so many years of thinking about my hair loss, I never really believed there was a possibility that all of my hair would fall out. When total hair loss finally happened, I felt relieved. (I did not realize this until I started writing this—sweet relief!) I didn't have to worry about what would happen next—it was done—or so I thought. Then the eyebrows and eyelashes started to go. Nobody told me this could happen! This was the first time I cried about my hair loss. Looking in the mirror I was no longer me—I was an alien from another planet. Waiting for my eyes to begin glowing green, I went to the internet to learn more about alopecia. I decided I needed to get my eyebrows and eyeliner tattooed on. I did this, thereby gaining the self-confidence to actually go out without wig or hat or scarf.

I found a number of support groups, made new friends and learned a lot about alopecia. There were so many people—5 million in the US alone—who are affected by this disorder. I took some comfort in the sheer numbers, but, if there were so many of us, why was it that no one seemed to know about it? Looking for a reason why, I decided that I lost my hair because I might be able to help someone else cope.

2004

My first outing au naturel was amusing and rewarding. I went to my friends' boutique. This was my home away from home and the safest place outside of my own house. This was always my first stop on a Saturday morning. I would visit, try on clothes and just hang out. These friends, a couple who are both artists, were

170

comforting and encouraging during my journey with alopecia. I wandered into the shop wearing a hat and quickly took it off. They both smiled and said I looked great. I had taken care to wear something feminine and top it off with some big funky earrings. Being a jewelry designer, I have more accessories than I know what to do with. I designed and made jewelry that was sold at the shop. I was becoming more comfortable with my oh-so-exposed head.

Suddenly, I spotted a woman with whom I worked. I was surprised to see her there. Though she had been to the shop before, it was not the norm to find her there. She gasped when she saw me.

I rubbed my head and said, "So how do you like my new do?"

Her eyes wide in wonder, she said, "You're not going to go to work like that, are you?"

Whew. I said, "Well, I don't think they are ready for it and it is obvious that you aren't, so I think I will wait a bit." End of discussion. My friends and I had a little chuckle and I survived.

A few minutes later, as I wandered through the racks helping customers as I often did, I encountered a lady who I did not know, but she looked at me as if I were familiar to her. I smiled and said, "Hello."

She quickly introduced herself to me and mentioned a friend we had in common. Then she blew me away. She thanked me for being brave enough to venture out without a head covering. She told me that she had alopecia and was so fearful that someone would find out. She had young children and was most afraid that other children would be unkind. We chatted for a long time. She thanked me again and told me that I had given her strength. I think I smiled until it gave me a headache! It was that moment that I knew why I had lost my hair. I have run into her a few times since then.

BOLDLY BALD WOMEN

2005

    I had been telling Jesse that he should get a tattoo on his head. He didn't seem to think that was a good idea, so I decided I should get one. Miami Ink, a tattoo reality show on The Learning Channel was fairly new and a big hit. Jesse told me his friends were on this show—he knew three of the artists on the show. The wheels started turning. I would get a tattoo on my head on this TV show and make a statement for my bald sisters and brothers. Back to the internet. Apply to get a tattoo on the show. Great. Sent them my story. Made a video talking about why I should be on the show. Weeks, maybe months went by.

    One day, I got a phone call from Miami Ink casting. They were actually considering me for the show. I think my son was surprised. More time went by as I spoke with more people and sent emails and pictures. It was an emotional roller coaster. By now, I had become a regular on the website: herhairlosshelp.com. I also met Dotty, who has a head full of tattoos. My friends encouraged me, but I began to doubt that I could pull it off. At last, the final phone call came from Miami Ink. I was going to film my episode on July 6, 2006. The artist I had requested for my tattoo was willing to do it!

    Next thing you know, we were on our way to Miami. I didn't think much about the process, just the fact that I was going to get my story out there! The casting folks were awesome, as were the production folks and the artists. A few days before the show was to air on October 2006, I emailed the local newspaper and asked them to consider doing a story on me, my tattoo and alopecia. To my surprise they phoned and said they would come to my house with a photographer. The next day—the day my show was to air—my bald head was on the front page of the paper—ME, the headline story! Must've been a slow news day. Between the news article and the TV show, I heard from hundreds of people who either had alopecia or were somehow affected by it.

2006 – 2008

Life goes on. I have had fun playing with wigs. A local wig store has become a place I like to visit. The owner and I have become friends. I find myself helping her to sell her wigs when I am there—even if I am not wearing one. I have met many lovely ladies with hair loss there and hope that I have helped some of them along the way. I spent the last few years wearing a wig to work and tossing it when I got home—or sooner, if the weather was warm. Since my first bald outing and after getting the tattoo, I have been spending the warmer months, outside of work, wigless.

2009

I attended my first NAAF conference in June 2009. I volunteered to help at the conference. My friend Dotty and I had the pleasure of facilitating a workshop—Dare to Be Bare. I knew that when I returned from the conference I would prefer to go to work without a wig. Summers in Boston can be rather warm and I needed to re-enforce my commitment. How could I tell people it was okay to be bald and then come back and hide my head at work? Of course, I was concerned that there could be problems. I had heard of people suffering discrimination because of their hair loss. Well, no such thing where I worked, thankfully. My friends and colleagues have been most supportive and complimentary. With the cold weather coming, I have taken to the wigs from time to time. It is nice to have options!

I have now been without hair for about six years. Attitudes and reactions to my appearance have both amused and annoyed me. There was the little kid at the mall who said, "Mommy, is that a boy or a girl?" My response was to stick out my chest and keep on trucking.

Then there was the guy who followed me through the supermarket talking about how beautiful bald women are.

I met a couple of big tough guys with shaved heads at a party a couple of years ago. They looked at my head with great envy. "Wow! What do you shave with?"

One of my favorites was a lady at my husband's high school reunion. She almost swallowed her tongue looking at me. I actually captured her expression on film—priceless.

I need to include a few words about guilt here. I must say that I have felt some guilt, because I did not experience the pain and anxiety that many women facing hair loss experience. I have even wondered if I had some basic deficiency because I managed to deal with my hair loss without a huge sense of personal loss. My total hair loss came at a time in my life when I was pretty much settled, secure and comfortable in my own skin. I must also mention that I have had amazing support. I now know, as a result of documenting my experience, that my strongest feeling after losing my hair was relief. It was the end of a long journey where this condition was chasing me. Although my hair finally did all fall out—I won. The chase was over. I am bald. So what?

Alopecia is now a big part of who I am in a positive way. My commitment to raising awareness and helping others has added purpose to my life. Several months ago, I joined with some friends to start a local non-profit to raise funds and awareness for alopecia. A few months ago, I filmed a local cable show talking about alopecia. In a few weeks, I will participate in a movie project dedi-

174

BOLDLY BALD WOMEN

cated to women and beauty. I will continue to boldly flaunt my
baldness and hope that the rest of the world can catch up with me!

—Joyce

❧❧

All I can say is, I rejoice in Joyce's lovely brazen spunk. I am grateful that alopecia gave me the impetus to seek her out. I am grateful to the website: AlopeciaWorld.com for enabling us to meet and form a friendship we are both certain will last through time and over all distance.

CHAPTER 17

Notes from Alopecians

꙰

TO DOCTORS

To know even one life has breathed easier because you have lived.
This is to have succeeded
—Ralph Waldo Emerson

꙰

Dear Doctors,

We know you are busy. We know you are pressured to keep to your schedule. We understand how hard you try to balance allotted time with patient needs, both physiological and psychological, including those patients trying to wrap their heads around the initial emotional trauma of hair loss. Cancer patients are prepared to expect hair loss before their chemo/radiation treatments begin. Alopecia can sneak up on a woman and, unless she is acquainted with the symptoms associated with the autoimmune disorder, it leaves her afraid and anxious.

I have included these notes from Alopecians for the purpose of providing physicians with a sampling of experiences and wishes of a small group of women from different countries. Although they express frustration, they mean no shame and blame. Some of these women have had their first experience with alopecia recently. Some have been dealing with it for forty years or more. Medicine has changed a lot in forty years, but the common themes of initial reactions to unexpected hair loss remain the same.

You will notice different beliefs as to the cause/triggers of alopecia. Although current research is promising, I must clarify that, at present, the cause of alopecia is unknown and there is currently no cure. I offer these comments as insight for you to assist your patients with their emotional responses to hair loss. It has often been said that alopecia is not life-threatening, but it is completely life-altering. The purpose of this book is to help women deal with the emotional aspects of female baldness. If only one of your patients benefits from something you learn from the comments below, you will fulfill my purpose. Information is the best tool any doctor has. Please, take whatever comments are helpful for you and leave the rest.

Sincerely,

Pam Fitros

෴

What advice did you initially receive from your doctors?

❖*My primary care physician and the first dermatologist I saw both told me my hair loss was due to stress, and if I removed myself from stress my hair would grow. The PCP did a whole series of blood tests to rule out thyroid disorder, lupus, hormone imbalance and many other possible diseases that could cause hair loss. My results were perfectly normal. I am as healthy as a horse! The specialist in alopecia areata I went to see told me stress is NOT the cause, though it may be a trigger.*

—Sandy K.

❖*My mother, sister and I had a major car accident in which we were hit by a drunk driver. Doctors at the time believed my nervous/immune system went haywire.*

—Faith

BOLDLY BALD WOMEN

❖ *It would be nice if doctors even knew what it was. Most do not and are also amazed by it.*

—Carol S.

❖ *Doctors have always said there is nothing they can do. It is still the same response. Before I fully understood this condition, I used to feel abandoned, as if it was insignificant. I now know the doctors are just as frustrated as I am because they are not to able to offer a cure.*

—Sharan

❖ *I was hopeful at first because she (the doctor) was. But I did my own research and I'm a realist. By the time I had several injection treatments, it was apparent to me it was not working. I think the doctor knew it wouldn't work and she informed me that my totalis presentation, ophiasis [a form of alopecia areata characterized by the loss of hair in the shape of a wave at the circumference of the head,] is most resistive to treatment. She monitored my process towards acceptance. That means that she stayed upbeat but not optimistic and allowed me to come to my own resolution to stop treatment.*

—Galena

❖ *I got very little advice. Doctors seem to know nothing about this disease.*

—Mary

❖ *I was disgusted. The GP [general practitioner] really didn't give me any confidence. I had to request certain tests to be carried out e.g., anemia and thyroid function et cetera. These results came back as negative. I then had to suggest/request a referral to a dermatologist. As time had moved on and the hair on my head was becoming pretty much non-existent, I decided to go privately to see the specialist, costing £100 (GBP). By this time, it was six months from the first appearance of a patch.*

The dermatologist confirmed alopecia and I quote, "What a shame

178

for a twenty-five-year-old. There is nothing we can do, because the hair loss is too extensive. It's a shame we didn't catch this sooner, as we could have tried steroids." I was very distraught at this time. From the hospital, I drove straight to one of my best friend's houses, and both my twin sister, Elin, and my friend, Melody, took the clippers to the remaining few clumps of hair. It was a traumatic but liberating experience.

—Gwennan

❖*My mother took me to several doctors, mainly dermatologists. We even visited the University of Michigan medical center. My diagnosis was alopecia areata. We were given some treatment options, including cortisone shots and intentionally sun burning my scalp among a few others. (The thinking behind the sunburn was that if the alopecia was an auto-immune problem perhaps the "attack" cells would be diverted to the sunburn instead of the hair follicles). Honestly, I can't even recall all of the treatments we tried, but I do remember that none of them worked. The doctors also told there us there was no specific cause of alopecia, but that it may be stress related and possibly auto-immune in nature.*

—Sarah

❖*My GP referred me to hospital for UV treatment. My loss was always too severe to consider steroid injections. At some appointments, many student doctors would be invited to see. That made me feel a bit of a guinea pig. There seems to be more awareness in the present day.*

—Sharan

❖*I have friends who are also doctors, and the amount of knowledge most doctors have about the various forms of alopecia is so minimal I have become my own advocate for what I need done.*

—Carol

In retrospect, what would have been most helpful to hear from your physician?

BOLDLY BALD WOMEN

❖ *The most helpful thing would have been honesty. To know that the doctors did not understand the condition fully and could NOT predict the outcome would have been very helpful. When I was about seven and had universalis, the dermatologist said it would never grow back. Then it all grew back a year later. Since then I have taken doctors' advice with a grain of salt. My alopecia started to get worse in 2004, but I have not been to see a dermatologist this time.*

—April

❖ *That I would be still be considered "beautiful."*

—Faith

❖ *"There is no cure for what you have, and no way to predict the course."*

—Mary

❖ *Just some advice and support. Rather than the utter lack thereof. Perhaps being offered counseling which, I retrospectively think, would have helped me through this tough time. Offering counseling should be standard. Perhaps suggestions of support groups, websites, books.*

—Gwennan

❖ *In retrospect, I wish my doctor would have said, "Kristine, you have Alopecia Areata, and there is no cure for it as of yet. It's just hair—your health is good otherwise. Find your inner beauty and just enjoy being you because life is short. Instead of wasting your money on hair potions and lotions that don't work, set that money aside and go on a trip someday!"*

—Kristine

❖ *The truth about alopecia, I guess. I didn't find that truth until I went to see the specialist nearly three months after the hair began falling out. I never did try any treatments, because the specialist I saw told me that it was unlikely the treatments would help over the long term.*

—Sandy K.

BOLDLY BALD WOMEN

❖ *How common it was. I felt isolated and alone and didn't see or meet anyone else with it so thought I was the only one. I was always spoken to as if it was rare.*

—Sharan

❖ *Frequently, fingernails may show dystrophic changes such as pitting, ridging, and thinning of the nail plate. When my fingernails went wonky, flaking off like mica (a silica mineral), my doctor had no idea why it was happening or what it was related to. The changes in my fingernails left me believing there was something more than just hair loss going on in my body. I needed to know that fingernail cells are just like hair cells, and it is common for fingernails and toenails to be involved with alopecia. Had my doctor told me it was part of the same auto-immune disorder, my anxiety would have dissipated.*

Also, it would have helped to know that Alopecians often have other autoimmune conditions, such as, allergies, asthma and eczema, and that a genetic component is common, although not always apparent.

—Pam

BOLDLY BALD WOMEN

Doctors provide us with information, possible treatment options, and sometimes help calm our fears and sooth our anxieties. It is
our families and friends who provide long term support and comfort
as we accept, assimilate, and grow through alopecia to a new self concept. Total baldness, such as that manifested in alopecia universalis,
changes the landscape of our self-perception. We look into the mirror
at a stranger and wonder what happened to the familiar face we used
to know.

My hair had been thinning and several spots were visible when
my husband left on an emergency trip to Greece because his mother
was gravely ill. By the time he came back two weeks later, most of my
body hair was gone. I had buzzed off the few remaining straggles of
mousy brown wisps and shaved my scalp smooth. I was wearing a wig
when I picked him up at the airport.

I watched Mike's tan face crease into crow's feet as he rolled his
carryon down the arrival ramp squinting and struggling to recognize
me with no eyebrows or eyelashes and topped by the wrong color
of hair in an unfamiliar style. He asked to see my head. I took the
wig off. I had prepared him on the phone, but hearing is different
from seeing. His moo cow brown eyes blinked several times, then
widened, arching the fine dark hairs of his eyebrows. I listened to
the sharp intake and long, slow exhale of his breath. Gentle fingers
explored my scalp.

BOLDLY BALD WOMEN

"It's as soft and smooth as a baby's butt," he said, his voice a breathy whisper accentuated by a heavy Greek accent.

I laughed, breaking the spell of his shock and wonder. He let go of his battered carryon bag and grabbed me in a bear hug. My Greek might be short, and getting older, but by gosh, he's as strong as an ox. He kissed me hard and whispered how much he missed me, a goofy grin on his face and a twinkle in his eyes.

As days went by he kept complaining to everyone who'd listen about how I was keeping him awake at night even after I'd finished reading and turned the book light out. Apparently, the moonlight streaming through our bedroom window was reflecting off my bald head and lasering his closed eyes with the glare. He figured we would never need a battery operated flashlight outside as long as there was moonlight and he could angle my head to shine in the direction in which he needed to see.

Mike amicably spoke of, gestured at, and joked about, my bald head. Those who were dumbfounded at my sudden baldness, and who were at a loss for words, didn't know whether to laugh or be horrified. Mike and I laughed and laughed at ourselves and my reflective head until the folks around us relaxed and understood laughter is not the enemy.

For me, hiding and secrecy are the sources of self-conscious discomfort, not my bald head. Mike's easy acceptance of my baldness, and his refusal to treat my bare head as the elephant in the room nobody talks about, helped me to be confident and casual about being bald. Don't think he hasn't held me while I cried over reactions of others to my alopecia, because he has, numerous times. But our Laurel and Hardy approach to life, finding whatever humor may be found in whatever situation we are presented with, works well for us. It has eased looking at and adjusting to the new skyline of my face for relatives and friends alike. It has helped us get through some pretty serious stuff over our forty-plus years together. But our way of coping is not for everyone.

Find what works for you and your Alopecian. The following notes are a mirror for family and friends of any woman dealing with hair loss to look into and see yourselves as you are, or, as you would like to be. Do you see yourself as an *encouraging* or *discouraging* force in your Alopecian's struggle to accept and love the new person she sees in her own mirror? Are you a comfort, or are you a knife in the fragile heart of her efforts to realign her self-esteem? You must find a way to be at ease with the change in your Alopecian if you are to help her be at ease with the change in herself. See how others have reacted and the affects those reactions had.

How did your family react to your hair loss?

❖ *They were alarmed, of course. My husband researched hair loss and came home one day with vitamin B supplements. My niece gave me several pre-natal samples from her job. I got so much advice from family members who knew I was losing my hair. I didn't share it with everyone in the family. After I shaved my head, my young son was frightened by my appearance and initially wouldn't let me hold him. My daughters were always great—very supportive. My middle child insisted that I come to the school bald for her scholastic awards program. I did and everyone at the school was supportive and kind.*

My parents are wonderful—Daddy said I looked like a model. Mommy is more matter-of-fact. My brother was ecstatic. He's bald and wanted to introduce me to his friends. My sisters are kind and encouraging.

—*Galena*

BOLDLY BALD WOMEN

❖ *My dad didn't say much about it. My mom was cruel and said that Kojack (Telly Savalas' popular TV show at the time) was my boyfriend. More support from my parents would have made a huge difference. I had one aunt who was very loving and supportive through it all. She had cancer and lost her hair. I knew that she understood. My husband of ten years has been completely supportive.*

—April

❖ *A distant relative said to me, "You're going to cover that thing (referring to my head) when we go outside, right?" I was so upset I cried and cried. I always felt very accepted at my in-laws' house. They didn't bat an eye even once if I got too hot and took off my hat or wig. They have always been wonderful.*

—Sandy K.

❖ *My son was only fourteen months old when I lost my hair, but my daughter was eight years old. She was as horrified as I was. I really think that my feelings about the hair loss, embarrassment, fear, and wanting to hide it, directly influenced her feelings about it too. She was by my side through everything and really experienced the changes right along with me. She was my rock! One of my favorite things happened when I first chose to go bald headed in public. We were at my son's tae kwon do school and my son (who was nine at the time,) came up behind me and pretended to polish my head with his shirt sleeve. People were shocked, but I laughed and laughed. Before long, we were all laughing.*

—Sandy K.

❖ *My family had their opinions and the painful ones were: "You shaved your head on purpose, just to be different. You're just doing it to prove a point. Oh no! Don't walk next to me. Yuck! You are completely bald. Go, go, go," a friend said to me while motioning to me with his waving hand to go away. I did walk away and never spoke to him again. "Now they will think you have cancer, so you* need to grow your hair *back." When I wore a wig: "Now you will look like a real woman. No, no! Don't take it off. I don't want you to spoil the good image I have of you." When I asked Mr. X which spectacles suited me: "How can I tell when you don't have hair?"*

Despite all the negatives, there have been people throughout the years who try to understand. My son said, "Losing your hair is nothing. It's not disfiguring and not worth crying over." I had one friend who has always said I'm beautiful without hair. One consolation!

—jO.

❖ *My parents and siblings were very protective of me. Especially because of the age that I was diagnosed (four years old.) Oftentimes I was isolated because of the newness of the diagnosis/disorder. Oftentimes I was kept from playing outside or from other outside activities because of the sun exposure and such.*

—Faith

❖ *My family is great. If I go to an event with a hat, they take it off and throw it so I can't find it. They love me and want me to be comfortable. My family gets life.*

—Carol S.

What did you want to hear from your family and friends?
❖ *What I did hear! That I am beautiful, with or without hair. I think my family's reaction made it so much easier. They all listened, supported, cared, and didn't feel they had to try to "fix" me. They love me no matter what, and they all showed me that throughout this process.*

—Sandy K.

❖ *That I was loved and that I was beautiful.*

—April

❖ *You still look beautiful. If showing your head is what you want to do, I still love you and approve of you and your choices.*

—Kristine

BOLDLY BALD WOMEN

❖*My aunt said, "You have always been pretty. I hate to say it, but you look GOOD bald!"*

—Carol S.

❖*I feel very accepted at church. The ladies of the church were the first people outside of my family to encourage me to be bald. They always tell me I'm beautiful. A Goldie Hawn look-alike at church swears that I'm sexy. She told me that real sexiness is more than hair. That was really nice because I think I'm unattractive. It's strange to embrace a new appearance and reconcile what you see with what others see.*

—Galena

❖*TAKE THE WIG OFF—YOU'RE BEAUTIFUL! There were people at church dealing with cancer and the radiation stages. The fact that I was bold enough to actually not put on my wig gave them encouragement to be free to be themselves.*

—Faith

What advice would you give to family members and friends of women newly diagnosed with alopecia?

❖*LISTEN! Don't try to make it better for someone who has just lost their hair, don't tell them about the latest hair replacement, or tell them to wear a hat, scarf, or wig. My mom listened to hours upon hours, upon hours, upon hours of hair talk. She is positively the best listener in the world! Be there to listen for as long as they want to talk about it. Let them know that they are beautiful and you love them hair—or no hair.*

My in-laws were terrific too. They didn't treat me any differently and were very open about asking questions and making sure I was comfortable in whatever situation. They were always very encouraging through the hair loss time and they continue to be that way today.

Oh, and when my hair was falling out, I was playing my trumpet in a jazz band. We had a concert coming up, and by the time the concert came, my hair was all gone. I was wearing hats all the time then. When

187

BOLDLY BALD WOMEN

I got to the concert stage, I noticed that ALL the trumpet players in the section were wearing hats too. I wasn't the only one wearing a hat. It really made me feel great that they were so supportive!

Some of my friends shrugged their shoulders and said being bald didn't matter. Others shied away from me as if alopecia were contagious. I found out who my TRUE friends were when I lost my hair.

—Sandy K

❖ *My mum's support was to always cover up. Don't be seen without my wig. This I found hard. I felt as if she was ashamed of me and I should cover up at all times. My sisters, too, gave me that impression. I was considering going to a job interview au natural. My sister commented that just because they were all used to seeing my bald head, didn't mean that everyone would be. This also made me feel as if I should conceal and cover up. It took me many years to put myself first, as my mum's view/support was quite detrimental to my acceptance of this condition. I wore a wig to make her feel better rather than it being for me. I wanted to know it was okay for me to be who I am. I would have come out a lot sooner if I had been reassured that, hair or no hair, it's okay to be who I am. Families and friends should help her maintain her femininity and identity. They should reassure her it is okay to be different. Get some specific support from people who understand.*

—Sharan

❖ *I could turn green in color all over and my friends would love me the same. I'm very blessed with the most beautiful friends one could wish for.*

—Kristine

❖ *My friendships didn't change in any way. They still love me. It was shocking at first, but I am okay with my baldness, so they became okay with it too. Quite often I forget I am bald because they don't act any different.*

—Carol S

188

BOLDLY BALD WOMEN

❖ *Tread lightly. Don't say trite things. Be supportive, be willing to listen. Let the grieving process take place. Relate to a family member with alopecia as a person beyond alopecia and help them to focus on other things.*

—April

❖ *Be there, but don't be overly sympathetic. Sympathy won't help. Offer possible solutions. When you lose your hair, you feel as though you are trapped and you have absolutely no idea where to go from here. They can help by working through options of whether wigs are right for you or not and supporting a decision to go bald. I definitely think getting good make-up advice would have been something I'd have found really helpful for learning tricks of how to conceal that you have no eyelashes/eyebrows. Clever make-up can be an instant and cheap boost to self-esteem.*

—Gwennan

❖ *Love and support her as best as you can. I'm talking about unconditional love and support. It is needed. Don't be afraid to talk about it. Tell her she still looks beautiful and if shaving her head is what she wants to do, you still love and approve of her and her choices. Shave your head in support and remind her that there is a lot more to do in life than to worry about loss of hair. Tell her to count her blessings—like the ability walk, talk, dance and sing, her health, and supportive friends and family.*

—Kristin

❖ *Support her and give her a shoulder to cry on. Give her acceptance. She has done nothing wrong to be where she is, just love her.*

—Carol S

❖ *Be loving. Be positive. Be there. Allow the Alopecian to grieve in her own way. Be aware of any mental issues that could arise and insist that she get counseling or join a support group.*

—Galena

BOLDLY BALD WOMEN

Do you love the woman in your life for who she is or for what she looks like?

If your answer is for what she looks like and you can't reconcile her bald head to your expectation of what your partner should look like, it's a real problem. Good long term sexual relationships happen when each partner feels loved, accepted, and cherished for who they are. Mind blowing sex in said relationship happens when both partners are confident they are attractive to their partner. If you find baldness unattractive, or down right disgusting, it is impossible to hide those feelings from your sexual partner. Unless you can come to terms with your reactions to her baldness, you can plan on a downward spiral in your sex life, or, if she acquiesces, condemn her to feel obligated to hide her true self under a wig or other head covering. It is not always the man's issue. Sometimes it is the woman's insecurity or self-loathing. Still, if you men aren't accepting and comfortable, it will be extremely difficult for a woman to be vulnerable and completely free in bed.

On the other hand, if you, like so many more men than I ever anticipated, find your lady's bald head to be exotic and sexy, you're home free.

❧

190

BOLDLY BALD WOMEN

❖ You know, the crazy thing is I think my hair falling out brought Marty (my boyfriend then, but husband now,) closer. I mean, he stayed by my side no matter what—and with the drastic change in my appearance—that was HUGE to me. He was amazingly supportive, and also a bit protective of me. He really wanted to shelter me from the mean people in the world. I had gone to an appointment with a specialist in alopecia and hair loss, fully believing that she would tell me that if I just take this medicine or that vitamin, my hair would grow back. However, after examining my scalp, she sank into her chair and said, "There is nothing I can do for you."

I was crushed, as I'm sure you can imagine, and I called Marty and told him what she said. His answer was, "You know what we should do? Let's go hat shopping!" He took me to this wonderful hat shop where we tried on every type of hat they had. He spent close to $300.00 on hats for me that day. Never once did he make me feel uncomfortable being bald. And even now when we go places, he is totally fine with my bald head. He makes me feel so beautiful all the time. I don't think I could be where I am today without his constant love and support.

—Sandy K.

❖ My last relationship was before my alopecia developed. Since my hair loss I hadn't had a boyfriend. Any guy I did meet was put off by my hair loss. Some were okay about it, but I never found anyone who loved me for who I was—until recently. I have met the most amazing and wonderful guy. He actually prefers me bald and he loves me for me. He's been a real pillar of strength. He has given me the courage and confidence to go bald, because he thinks I'm beautiful without hair.

—Gwennan

❖ I was telling a college friend yesterday that I feel bad because this guy was checking me out on campus and I think he's cute. I doubt *that I would have gotten that attention if I was still bald. And I think the fallacy there is that I don't get the attention during those times when I am completely bald because I doubt. I have definitely felt unattractive because of my alopecia, but, at the end of the day, it is a huge part of who I am. It has made me who I am today, as much as I would initially have hated to admit that. I don't know who I would be without alopecia. I can't even fathom that.*

—Caitlin

❖ *I guess my anxiety and depression made me feel less sexual, but my husband still desires me as much as he did before the hair loss.*

—Galena

❖ *I keep a bandanna on even in bed. It is hard for me to be totally uncovered and not feel unattractive.*

—April

❖ *I take my makeup off at night, and don't like my partner to see me without eyebrows and eyeliner, but my partner lets me know how gorgeous he thinks I am all the time without hair.*

—Carol S.

❖ *The first thing my husband did after our wedding was shave his head. Since then he has never gone out without it being cleanly shaved. He tells me daily that I look beautiful.*

—Willow

❖ *My husband, Cliff, made coping with alopecia easier. He helped me out by running the first clipper buzz across my head in my moment of indecisiveness on whether I should shave my head or not. After he did that the room filled with silence. We just stared at each other as we looked at each other in the mirror with the biggest smiles on our faces. We were both at a loss for words. There was no turning back. He finished shaving my head and then he kissed me on the head and told me he loved it! My*

BOLDLY BALD WOMEN

shaved head totally turned Cliff on. He's a big Trekkie fan and suggested that all I needed now were the pointy ears. Grrrrr. I thought, how lucky am I? Cliff has made living with alopecia areata so easy for me with his unconditional love. He told me the other day, "Babe, if you ever are able to grow your hair back, will you please still shave it?" I LOVE HIM!

—Kristine

BOLDLY BALD WOMEN

꙳

TO EMPLOYERS AND CO-WORKERS

What you leave behind is not what is engraved in stone monuments,
but what is woven into the lives of others.
—Pericles

꙳

Do you remember the story about Samantha, whose employer told her she was no longer acceptable to represent his office because of her weight and recent baldness? Samantha is not alone in her experience of discrimination and harassment.

꙳

❖ *Initially, I was so shocked and embarrassed by my hair loss that I wanted to wear hats. The company I was working for insisted that, if I were to wear a hat, it had to be one of the company hats with the company logo. Well, the company hat was a baseball style cap with a mesh back. Everyone could see my bald patches through the mesh. It was humiliating and depressing all at the same time. What got me most in that job was that as my hair fell out my co-workers began to treat me differently. I mean, it was a vending company (filling vending machines) and I was the office manager. The people that ran routes and filled the machines often needed me to refill their coin bags and sometimes needed their route plans changed around. Before I lost my hair, they would come to me without any problem, tell me what they needed, and go about their business. But the more that my hair fell out, the more they treated me as if I were stupid! They began to speak slowly and over-enunciate their words as if, by losing my hair, I had forgotten English or something. I remember one time a woman was speaking slowly to me and then asked 'Do—*

194

you—un—der—stand?' I was so fed up with being treated like this that I slammed my hand on the desk and hissed through my teeth, "Look! I know that I may look stupid, but I'm NOT stupid, okay?' She rolled her eyes and said "Whatever," and stormed out.

Anyway, I quickly (thankfully) found a new job in a retail establishment running their cash office, and left the vending company. Since then, the vending company has gone out of business, so my timing in leaving was actually very good. Ha! I am now a realtor, and no, I do not wear hats to work. If the weather is chilly I will wear a scarf, or sometimes a hat while outside, but if I get too hot—off it goes.

—Sandy K.

❖ *I got fired because I was fighting for my rights against discrimination. I was being held back because of my appearance. Although it was acceptable in the company policy for associates to wear a baseball hat with a company logo on it, I was somehow an exception to that rule.*

I was furious at the news of an Owen Sound woman who shaved her head for cancer. She was asked to take the summer off with her kids so her hair could grow out. The restaurant owner described her appearance as "appalling."

—Carol J.

❖ *The stares from co-workers and the whispers. People thought I was lying about why I was going bald. Having to explain non-stop got to be too much. Some of my co-workers are the most immature people I had to deal with. I would not wish them on anyone. It was only a handful, but that handful was enough. One day, coming home from work, I was crying so hard. I was wearing a bandana and had nothing else to wipe my eyes with and blow my nose on, so I took the bandana off my head, cried into it, and then blew my nose. And no, I did not put it back on my head. That was my first bald experience. It was kind of cool and I laughed really hard. I must have looked like a crazy bald chick laughing to herself.*

—Carol S.

❧

Company policies must include protection for bald women from discrimination, and make certain all employees attend an in-service about what alopecia is and how to act appropriately towards a woman with alopecia. There should be zero tolerance for harassment and discrimination, overt or covert. Her bald head does not change a woman's ability to do her job. It is only the discriminatory harassment, subtle or not so subtle, by co-workers that affects her job performance.

If you, the Alopecian, or someone you know with alopecia is being harassed or discriminated against at work, find out what steps need to be taken to correct the situation.

❖ Start by going to the human resources department.

❖ If that doesn't work, go to the local labor board.

❖ It may even mean having to call upon the investigative team of the local TV station and taking the company to task publicly.

It's not likely you'd get your job back, and, if you did, there is still a possibility your work environment could remain hostile. But at least the company might think twice about doing the same thing to the next woman working for them who experiences hair loss.

❧

THE CANCER QUESTION

❧

I like getting The Cancer Question because I can answer, "Yes, I'm an ovarian cancer survivor, but that's not why I'm bald." Conversations get started that way that end up in the strangest places. I was perusing packaged meat in the local grocery store, you remember—the regular grocery stores before the advent of Costco, Sam's Club and Walmart superstores. They are almost extinct now. Still there I was looking at the meat, when a Very Pregnant woman waddled up next to me and began to bemoan the cost of ground chuck beef. She asked me if I was having chemo treatments and I gave her the standard educational answer and then I asked when she was due to deliver and if this was her first child.

"No," she said, cupping her belly gently with work worn hands, "this is my sixth child and I am due any minute now."

I scrunched one eye and cringed. "Any minute now? So, what are you doing looking in a grocery store at 10:00 PM muttering over the price of hamburger?"

"Oh! Not hamburger—never hamburger," she said in a voice tainted with shock. "My husband and I have a farm and we raise grass fed Angus beef for ourselves and to sell. We are very careful about the quality of meat we eat. And this stuff," she said, her face crinkled in disgust and her slender arms gesturing at the lumps of meat in Styrofoam containers tightly wrapped with clear cellophane, "well, this stuff was fed with...you don't want to know what that steer was fed or even if it was an old cow that didn't give much milk anymore. And look at the price! It's exorbitant!" She brushed back a strand of chestnut hair that had dislodged from her pony tail and fallen into her face.

"We've run out of our winter supply of meat and the next steer won't be ready for slaughter until next week. I had to come to town today for an appointment with my doctor and thought I'd visit my sister at the same time. Now I'm on my way home and I need some ground beef for tomorrow's supper." She took a breath and her blue eyes winced as a pronounced bulge poked out from the left side of her belly and slammed her several times in rapid succession.

"Tell me you're not going to have that baby in the meat aisle of this D & W grocery store," I said anxiously.

"Nope. This one's not coming tonight—but he sure is getting testy all squashed up in there." She chose a family-sized package of ground beef and angled her gianormous belly toward me. "Well," she said, "it was nice chattin' with you. It's time me and this baby are headed home. We've got a forty-five minute drive ahead of us to get out of the city and back to the farm."

"Wait a minute," I said, "Do you have a business card? I'd be interested in getting a quarter of beef at the end of the year if you have enough"

She pawed around in her purse and shook her head, dislodging the strand of hair again. "No, I guess I forgot to replenish my supply after I used the last one."

"I can't imagine how you might have forgotten," I said and snickered. "Five and nine-tenth kids and a mini cattle ranch—not much else on your plate, right?"

She pushed the uncooperative hair clump over her right ear. "You got it. Well, I've got a piece of paper and a pen right here, so I'll write it all down for you."

And she did. And I smacked that piece of paper to my refrigerator door with a heavy-duty, checker-sized magnet and kept it there where I wouldn't forget where I'd put it.

And that's how alopecia and The Cancer Question got me a freezer full of the best beef I've tasted since I was a little girl when my Mama made us Sunday roast beef with onions, carrots and potatoes nestled around it and cooked until they were tender and browned. She'd top everything off with her marvelous gravy. That was some mighty good eatin'.

BOLDLY BALD WOMEN

Yes, I love The Cancer Question! Here are some other experiences with TCQ.

❦

❖ *Oh, yes! I'd get TCQ (The Cancer Question) every day. It used to bother me when people would mistake me for a cancer patient. I am NOT sick! I don't think I look sick, I'm just hairless. But then it dawned on me one day that, when people ask, it's usually because they have either gone through chemotherapy themselves, or they know someone who has, and they are really looking to provide support and encouragement. I finally learned to say, "Oh, thankfully no. I'm not sick. I have alopecia areata. Basically, my hair just doesn't grow." Sometimes I go into more detail with what I call, Alopecia 101, but not always. It depends on my mood. I guess I really want people to feel free to ask about my hairlessness, but please don't assume I'm sick.*

—Sandy K.

❖ *People ask if I'm going through chemo and ask what stage of cancer I'm in. I've also had people question my sexuality. It's just absurd. I would never ask a stranger these questions.*

—Kristine

❖ *Sometimes I correct people and give them one of my alopecia awareness cards. Other times I accept the empathy and keep moving on.*

—Galena

❖ *Any time I have been asked the cancer question, I tell them about alopecia, and they are probably sorry they asked because I give lots of detail about alopecia. Not everyone who is bald is sick. Not all women who are bald need to be pitied. Some of us have grown to enjoy the bald look.*

—Carol S.

❖ *I'd like to see awareness reach an acceptable level so that we are not labeled immediately as poorly with cancer. It's a difficult label to get rid of and people should know more than this one-way street.*

—Sharan

❖ *We still have a long way to go before people stop assuming we're chemotherapy patients or understand that bald can be attractive too. That is why I will always do everything possible to put us on the fast track to awareness and acceptance.*

—Carol J.

᷆᷆᷆

THOUGHTFUL THINGS TO SAY OR DO

᷆᷆᷆

If you really want to know what to do and how best to do it, get the answers from the source.

❖ *When I finally, after eight years of living with alopecia, put the wigs away and decided to go out bald-headed, I went to the library. One of the staff working there said hello to me and told me I was totally rockin' the bald look. I was so happy because, quite honestly, I didn't think I could pull off the bald look!*

—Sandy K.

❖ *It is better to be asked an honest question and have a chance to tell my story than to be STARED at. Please understand that alopecia is an ongoing thing. Some days I am more accepting of my condition than others and those days feel like there is a purpose to what I'm going through. More than anything I want to be normal again, but, if I'm going to continue to deal with this, I want there to be a way that my experiences can help someone.*

—April

BOLDLY BaLD Women

❖ *I am still a human being like everyone else. Accept that people are different. Don't make generalized assumptions. Taking a tactical approach always helps.*

—Gwennan

❖ *I have been told by strangers that I do the bald thing well.*

—Carol S.

❖ *I have been hugged and told, "thank you" for being brave to encourage and educate.*

—Faith

❖ *Send pretty bandanas, compliment her, and notice when she is having a bad day.*

—April

☙〜❧

THINGS TO AVOID SAYING OR DOING

☙〜❧

Pay close attention to this list of don'ts unless you want to find yourself having to deal with jumping on your Alopecian's last nerve. Standing on a live wire is not the smartest place to be in a rainstorm, so head's up and eye's sharp to avoid emotional electrocution—her's and your's.

☙〜❧

❖ *Don't talk with others about my alopecia unless I have given you permission to do so.*

—April

❖ *STARING! It is okay from little kids, because I expect that from them, but not from adults. Sometimes they get so caught up in staring at the bald chick in the room, that when I say hello to them, or smile, they don't even notice. That really bugs me!*

One time I was shopping for clothing and a strange woman came

201

up to me from across the room. In a very harsh tone, she said, "My God! What happened to your hair?" I admit I wasn't kind as I matched her tone of voice and replied, "Nothing! What happened to your hair?" She smacked her lips, turned on one heel, and walked away. Immediately after saying that, I felt bad for being so rude, but, looking back now, it was kind of funny.

—Sandy K.

❖ The staring game. My eyes are bigger and I will always win.

—Faith

❖ There is a big difference between an inquisitive look and one of either pity or disgust.

—Carol J.

❖ Teachers, don't single out bald children as being one of the special abnormal kids. I was in the first grade when I lost my hair completely. I thought I was ugly and became withdrawn. I excelled in academics and tried to be a helper to my teachers. I kept to myself and trusted a few close friends. Kids' remarks at school, having things thrown at my head on the playground were insensitive and hurtful.

—April

❖ Don't push me to wear a wig when I don't want one. My mom, who also has alopecia and rocks her wigs, was persistent about my needing to buy a wig. We would spend time together going out for coffee, running errands and shopping. Somehow, we always ended up with Mom pulling into the wig shop parking lot, and begging me to try on all the wigs. It was the fastest way to sour a great day together. I know my mom was just looking out for me. She wanted to protect me from anyone saying rude things. The love my mom has for me is immeasurable, but she had no idea how confident a woman she raised. I just don't care to wear a wig.

—Kristine

BOLDLY BALD WOMEN

❖ *Don't ask me anything about being bald. Just compliment me on my avant garde fashion sense.*

—*Galena*

❖ *Don't express envy about my ability to just shake my hair (wig) and plop it on my head in the morning. It grates on my last nerve!*

—*April*

❖ *Please don't pity me because you could be talking to someone who embraces her baldness and has no problem with it. Someone who, in fact, loves being bald. Life is short and we should live each day as if it is our last. I don't want to leave this planet Earth knowing my final concerns were about my hair. Right now I'm into forgiving myself for all of the shame I put on myself over the years resulting from alopecia areata. I am still feeling like a beautiful woman.*

—*Kristine*

❖ *I so dislike being mistaken for a bloke. If I'm not dressed feminine, I'm automatically assumed to be a bloke.*

—*Sharan*

❖ *Nothing happened when I was out bald that tore me down. I did hate going through the mall on Saturdays. Saturday is the teen promenade day. Young folks snickered, laughed and stared at me the whole time. I vowed never to shop at the mall on Saturday again without a head covering. Although people haven't said anything rude or tactless, I felt the why-doesn't-she-wear-a-scarf-or-hat non-verbal communication from a woman once. My baldness was making her uncomfortable, so I stared at her until she walked away. I'm very intuitive about others reactions, but their reactions have nothing to do with my emotional process.*

—*Galena*

BOLDLY BALD WOMEN

༻✦༺

TRANSFORMATIONS, GEMS OF WISDOM

༻✦༺

And the Good News is…

❖ *All my fears are gone. When I was younger my fear was that my hair would never come in. Now I know it probably won't ever come in and I'm okay with that. I would probably be scared if it starts to come in again. I don't want partial hair, as I am so at peace now. I hardly consider or think about my loss anymore. Since coming out I'm not consumed with the process of concealment and covering up—which can take over your life and existence. I accept that I can't accept I have alopecia. Sounds daft, but it works for me. I think others see me as more patient, calm and assertive with how I have coped with my challenges. I am not so quick to judge others. I feel proud of myself, having come through such a difficult journey and survived. I have such a passion to support others with this affliction as I feel I was far too isolated with very little support.*

I am at a place I never felt I could reach in my life. I am not embarrassed about my hair loss, neither am I ashamed of my alopecia. I am on a very different platform now where the view is amazing. I have boxed away my worries and anxieties from the past and I have moved on to a brighter place where I keep my thoughts positive. This results in actions and beliefs being positive. These positive things bring opportunity towards your life. Doors open that you never knew were there. I don't know if the trauma I went through as a young girl has resulted in my life without hair. I will never know the answers to some questions, but I won't dwell on that. I will move on with courage and determination.

—Sharan

❖ *Coping with alopecia has allowed me to understand the depth of my strength and courage. It has allowed me to build a stronger foun-*

204

dation with myself, my self-image and my confidence. I am a work in progress, ready to blaze trails not yet taken, while educating, promoting awareness, and enhancing the beauty of being a BEAUTIFUL ALO-PECIAN.

—Faith

❖Wigs are uncomfortable, hot, itchy and I like being bald. I do find some women to be very gorgeous bald, that's what gorgeous earrings are for, and lots of eye makeup. I have never been huge on makeup, but now I keep them in business. I don't like the fact I do not have eyebrows and eyelashes. I can handle being bald, and really kind of like it, as I never have been someone who likes to fuss with her hair, and, at times, found it to be a pain in the ass. But I do miss the loss of defining hair for my eyes. Men have strived to have the comfort level of being bald for themselves. I do the bald look so it becomes an option for me and other gals. I definitely look different to myself, but I am not one to ever slam myself—it serves no purpose to me. Now I look at myself as a pretty bald chick. I'm not saying I don't cry still, because I do. But I do it a whole lot less. There are days when I get bummed thinking that my head hair might grow back, because I have grown to enjoy looking different. People used to say, "Oh, you look so much like so-and-so." I don't get that any longer. I have my own look now.

—Carol S

❖I hope greater interest will be taken in childhood alopecia and that children will have a cure, because I believe it is harder for children who get it. As women we have stronger minds and can deal better with it.

—Carol S

❖It is an emotional roller coaster of transformation—learning to accept our new image, self-worth and way of living in confrontation with our *Self* and others. *Call it enlightenment of sorts. I am embarking on a new journey, leaving my past in the past, on to a new fresh path, a new future, a new way of living and loving myself. Let's strive to create an awakening of the minds. The minds of our fellow human beings who lack the knowledge, understanding, empathy and compassion to accept people with alopecia.*

—jO

❖ *It's been a journey. I was beautiful when I had hair, and, now I can say I feel beautiful not having hair too! Shortly after I shaved my head, I got a beautiful, colorful tattoo of a butterfly on the left back side of my neck. It is very symbolic to me of my metamorphosis while living with alopecia. It is a daily reminder that I AM BEAUTIFUL STILL.*

—Kristine

❖ *My friends, family and I try to make light of my alopecia. Not to make a joke about it, but to try and take it at face value and turn what has happened into a positive. My boyfriend used to put my old wig on, which always made me laugh! My nephew likes to slap (gently, might I add) my bald head, which makes him and me crease with laughter. I joke that one day I'm going to walk into a hair salon and ask for a perm!*

—Gwennan

❖ *I love feeling the wind blow over my scalp during the hottest days in South Carolina. Before going bald I only felt the sweat running down underneath my wigs.*

—Faith

❖ *At first I was so heartbroken. At times I did think of taking my life because of the pain that people had caused me at work. The isolation that hair loss in a woman causes can be too much. I would just like to make life for women going through physical changes as accepted as it is*

206

BOLDLY BALD WOMEN

for men—hair loss, weight gain, aging—whatever it is, women need to be loved just like men when they go through their physical changes. We can't always be twenty-year-old models.

—Carol S.

❖ *I am Gwennan, with or without hair. It's what's inside that matters. I am very lucky to have a fantastic family, a great group of friends and an amazing boyfriend, who all see me for who I am. I have got to where I am because of who I am. I try to remind myself that a lot of people would have given up and hidden away. Having a fighting and uncompromising spirit, I have never wanted to let anything or anyone hold me back. This spirit was trodden on but somehow, with the support of a lot of people around me, has shone through.*

—Gwennan

❖ *In spite of starting off with alopecia feeling sad, scared, and embarrassed to be bald, I write to you today happy, strong, and proud to be the person I am. I am boldly, happily, uniquely bald. Alopecia universalis has not been the end, but a brand new beginning for me. And, joy really does return in the morning! Life is good—hair or no hair.*

—Sandy K.

❧❦

EPILOGUE

What's Blowing in the Wind
Now that my Hair Isn't?
ै✺✫

The answer, my friend, is blowin' in the wind.
The answer is blowin' in the wind.
—Bob Dylan

✺✫

I breathe a sigh of relief. And then another of regret. Boldly Bald Women is as complete as I can make it. Finished. I have created a stepping stone on the path to acceptance of female baldness in a society conditioned to infatuation with women's hair. But there is a niggle in my mind I can't put a name to. It keeps telling me I've missed something.

Then I watched an episode of Parenthood on NBC TV. It is entitled: *Keep on Rowing.* The episode deals with the reaction of a main female character to losing her hair as a result of chemotherapy. What was this? Female baldness on prime time TV?

Beautifully told, the story line catches the emotions of the first clump of errant hair falling onto the restaurant table during a girls' night out celebration of the successful lumpectomy to remove our heroine's breast cancer. The celebration stops, replaced by silent horror and acute embarrassment. Fear wells up in widened eyes. Fleeting glances flash from one woman to another as the clump of lifeless hair is strategically removed from sight. Everyone scrambles for words of comfort. The party is over.

Our heroine goes home to a sleeping household to face her reality in the mirror. With tears, half smiles and quivering lips she uses her husband's electric shaver to buzz her head and follows that with a close razor shave. With one last look in the mirror and a flicker of hope in her eyes, she moves quietly to her dark bedroom and taps her sleeping husband on his arm, hopefulof his understanding and support for her courage.

"I did it," she says, shaking him into wakefulness.

"Did what," he mutters more asleep than awake. He opens one eye to look at his wife.

The next scene shows him wide awake, jumping out of bed, fumbling for the table stand light and shouting, "What the..." The look on his face when the light comes on makes it clear he thought his wife's shaven profile was an alien bending over him in the dark.

That creates a dissonance between them that worsens as he tries to rectify his initial reaction. He buys her a wig when he sees her looking at wigs on the internet. She over-reacts to his gesture believing that he thinks she is ugly rather than just trying to help.

The next day she shows up at his job, having set up a surprise for him with the help of his assistant—a night at a great hotel and a date as husband and wife instead of husband and cancer patient. Pat, pat, kiss, kiss, hug, hug and all is well, except that she loses her strength and must sleep instead of reveling with him

The following morning they are dressed and leaving their room for checkout. We see him in an impeccable suit, pulling the wheeled overnight case into the hallway. He stretches his hand toward the open room door and we see our heroine's hand take his as she moves into the hall. She is dressed in chic winter white pants and a gorgeous white coat belted with black. Her head is bald. She is beautiful. She is confident. Her husband looks at her adoringly. She lifts her head and they stroll toward the front door of the hotel. The limousine waits at the entrance. Her husband opens her door and our heroine slides in gracefully. He follows her in. The limousine pulls regally away and the scene fades.

I'm sitting quietly on the couch in the family room, tears sliding down my face. I feel proud. I am proud that the subject of female baldness has been approached on national television in a prime-time slot in such a thoughtfully encompassing presentation. I'm proud that our heroine found her way to her self, and her husband to acceptance of and pride in his wife's new beauty all in just one episode. The only thing that could have made it better would have been if the actress actually shaved her own head. The bald prosthetic covering her hair made her head look disproportionately large and more science fiction than true life. Still, the impact of total hair loss was well presented.

The niggle in my mind telling me I am missing something grows more insistent.

Then one of my Alopecian friends tells me about an episode of HBO's *Sex and the City, An American Girl in Paris, Part One.*

I watched the sound bite (http://www.youtube.com/watch?v=nKvTlXgsb80) and see a woman having a post chemo hot flash standing at a podium in a room full of women. The women are there for an inspirational speech about dealing with cancer. Finally, the speaker, now dripping with full body sweat, can't stand the wig on her head another minute. She tears it off while making a joke about her make up dripping down her face. She looks down to wipe the sweat from her chest and fans herself with her wig. When she looks back up, a bald woman stands with her wig in her hand. Another woman rips off her wig and stands. The whole room erupts into applause as every woman wearing a wig to cover her hair loss takes off the wig and stands to show the speaker she is not alone.

I'm crying again, while I applaud with them. I've been there. I've seen my makeup slowly run down my face. I've been hot too, not from chemo because I never had any for my own bout with ovarian cancer. My poor Alopecian scalp overheated from the wig itself—but my misery matched that of the speaker's sweaty drop for sweaty drop.

The niggle remains. What am I missing?

Mary Marshall sent me an email telling of her newest idea. She calls it The Bald Mannequin Project™. Mary is asking bald women to go to department stores that display bald mannequins and have themselves photographed in model poses next to the mannequins. The object is for Mary to create a collage display on Facebook of the real bald women of the world.

Says Mary, "For a long time, it's bugged me that so many of the mannequins in fashionable stores are bald, whereas real bald women are rarely seen and certainly not used by the fashion industry. Besides showing the world what real bald women look like, we can show the world what normal-size women look like next to the mannequins! If FAKE bald women are the height of beauty and glamour, why can't REAL bald women be too?"

I laugh, thinking what a wonderful idea this is. And I imagine all the pictures bald women will send to Mary of themselves having fun standing next to those elegant bald mannequins going viral on the internet. A bell chimes inside my thoughts. *Ding, ding, Pam! HERE IT IS! THIS IS WHAT YOU MISSED.*

This book begins with an invitation to a train ride—a journey to understanding, acceptance, and hope for those women who, for what ever reason, got off the Life Train at the same station I did: Bald Boulevard.

BOLDLY BALD WOMEN

A train ride has a predetermined track with expected stations and stops. When I started writing this book I thought Boldly Bald Women would be another piece of track laid down on a line of expected, predictable and hard won mechanical progress away from the Bald Boulevard Station headed towards Acceptance Avenue Station.

But somewhere along the way, Boldly Bald Women is blowing a vigorous wind of change. Women are embracing the possibilities of being Boldly Bald from the shared stories of their sisters, and soaring with them. These ideas gather momentum, take flight, morph into more ideas that ride the thermal-currents generated by the ideas themselves, crossing continents and cultural chasms of ideology and prejudices with a determination, vigor and grace. I did not, could not have imagined the possibilities in the beginning of this writing.

My sisters, my friends, those of you I have wrapped in heartfelt hugs, and those of you I have not yet met, and perhaps never will meet—we're not on a train ride anymore. We're flying! Every difficulty faced, every wrong exposed and righted, every story shared, every bald head courageously and proudly bared, gives another bald woman wings of hope, wings of courage. Fly, my sisters—whatever the reason for your baldness, whatever the season in your life—fly and soar to become who you are—the Boldly Bald Women of the World!

My love and joy flies with you,

Pam Fitros

One Boldly Bald Woman shining among many.

Pam Fitros

∿◦∾

"This is me, post ovarian cancer. I did not lose my hair, as I had neither chemo nor radiation therapies.

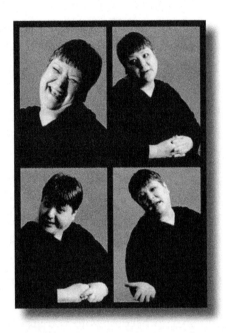

"These are my emergence photos. We bald women have to put on our big girl panties and clothe ourselves in humor and compassion to shield us from initial shock reactions of others. Give people time and be patient. Remember how shocked you were when you saw yourself bald for the first time."

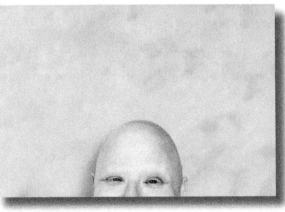

BOLDLY BALD WOMEN

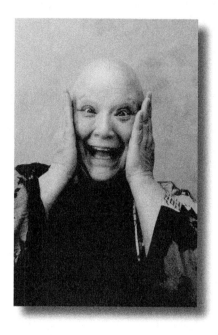

"Ready or not, here I come!"

"Now I ask you, what's not to love?"

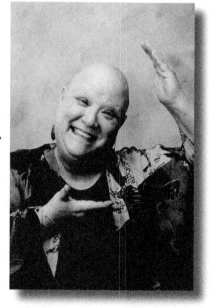

BOLDLY BALD WOMEN

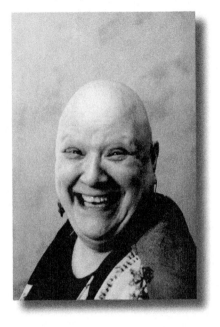

"This new look rocks!"

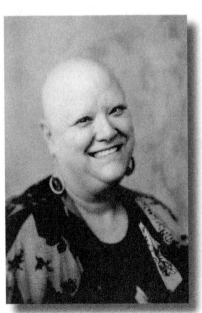

"Well, here I am, the new me. A Boldly Bald Woman. I love it! The only hair I miss is my nose hair. Nose hair filters air, warming it in winter and keeping pollen and bugs out in summer. Nobody really appreciates nose hair—until it isn't there."

BOLDLY BALD WOMEN

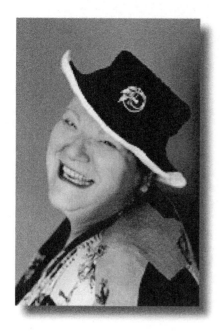

"My sister's hats."

"I am blessed to have a talented sister who loves me big. I know that because it takes many hours and patience to make each hat and she made me gazillions.

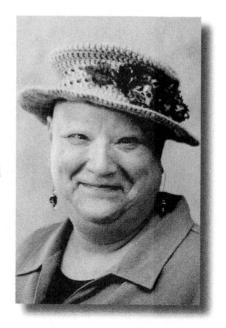

BOLDLY BALD WOMEN

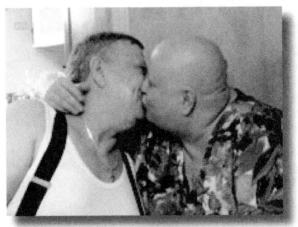

"The Greek and I.
As Abraham Lincoln once said,
'People are just as happy as they make up their minds to be.'
Life is what you make it. We choose to live it in happiness and gratitude
for each new day we have together."

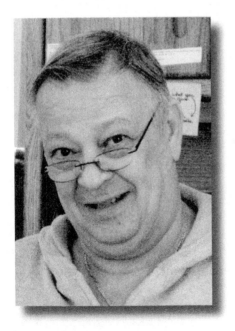

"Hrisostomos Fitros (aka Mike The Greek), my husband, my best friend, the love of my life. The man who keeps forgetting I don't need shampoo anymore when I shower, just soap. My wonderful Little Greek, who has sacrificed above and beyond to enable Boldly Bald Women to become a reality."

aLOPECia WORLD

❧

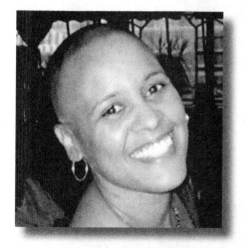

"Cheryl Carvery-Jones came up with the idea of Alopecia World."

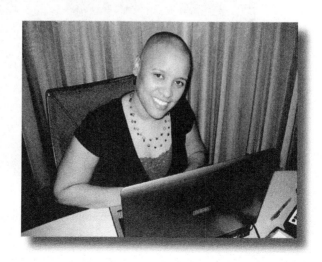

BOLDLY BALD WOMEN

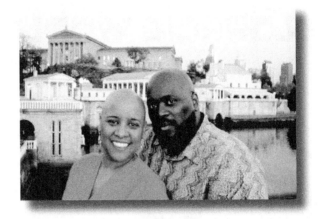

"Cheryl and RJ co-founders of Alopecia World."

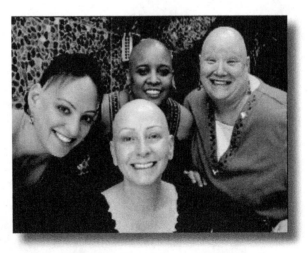

"Caitlin, Cheryl, Pam, and Meg
working together to raise alopecia awareness."

InternatIonal alopecIa Day

⊰∘⊱

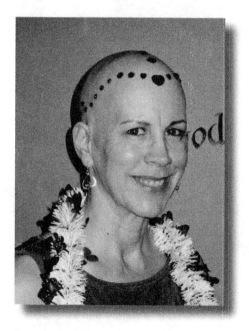

"Mary Marshall, creator and coordinator of
International Alopecia Day™."

BOLDLY BALD WOMEN

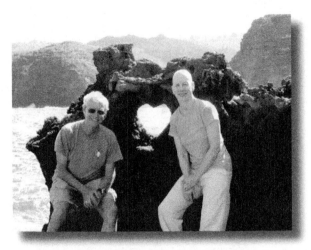

"Mary and husband Steve Gould, internationally known photographer."

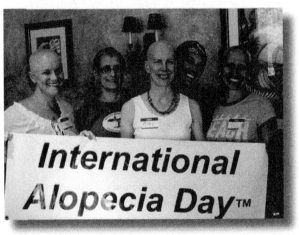

"Some of the participants in the San Diego IAD celebration. Left to right, Jessica Smith, Linda Timlin, Mary Marshall, Elena Martinez, and Teresa Hill Flannery."

BOLDLY BALD WOMEN

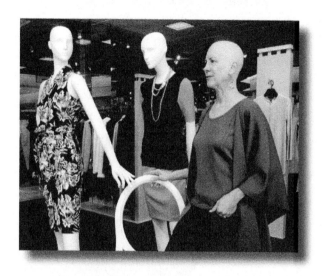

"Mary's new idea, The Mannequin Project™."

OLIVIA RUSK

❧

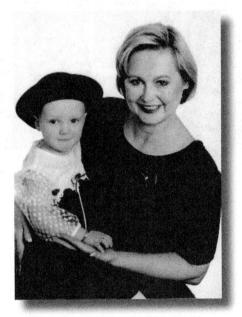

"Olivia as a baby."

BOLDLY BALD WOMEN

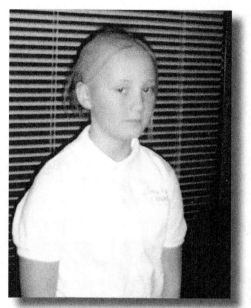

"Olivia's hair fell out for the second time."

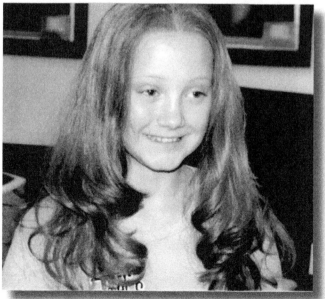

"Olivia had an opportunity to get a custom made Farrel human hair vacuum wig."

BOLDLY BALD WOMEN

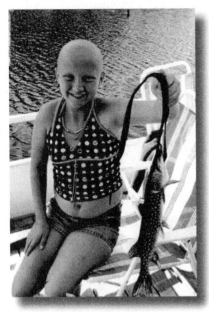

"Olivia decided she didn't like the heat and hassle of gluing the vacuum wig to her head and has never worn another."

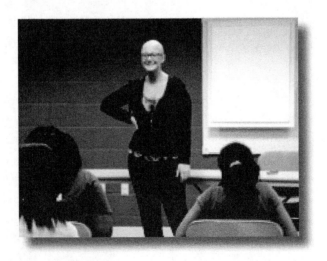

"Olivia begins speaking to young audiences around the country."

BOLDLY BALD WOMEN

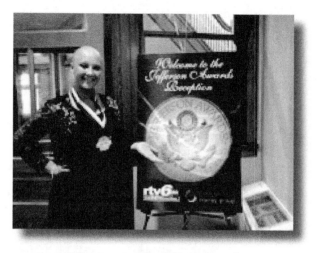

"Olivia receives the Jefferson Award.
Local winners are 'Unsung Heroes'— ordinary people
who do extraordinary things without expectation of recognition."

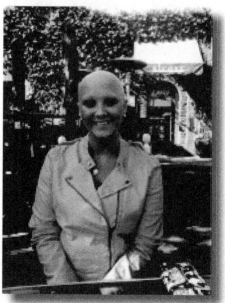

"Olivia at fourteen years old. I can't wait to see what her future holds! See her on
Olivia's Cause in Facebook and visit www.oliviascause.org"

JOYCE BRIER

☙❧

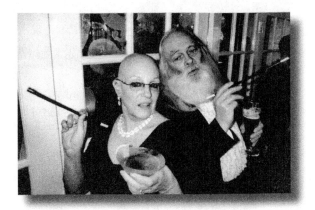

"Joyce and Walt Brier."

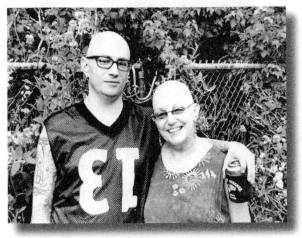

"Joyce and her son, Jessie, who has alopecia too."

BOLDLY BALD WOMEN

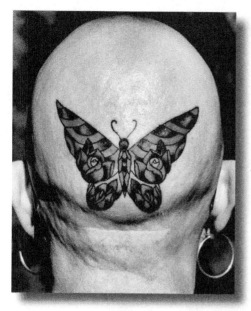

"Joyce had her head tattooed on the TV program Miami Ink. She says her butterfly tattoo is a great conversation starter and helps her get the message out about alopecia. You can see the video on YouTube at: http://www.youtube.com/watch?v=zTxSDftIEdA"

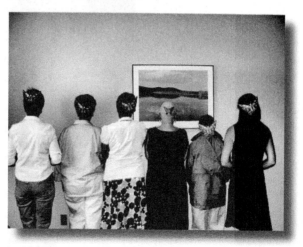

"Joyce's co-workers all had plastic butterflies clipped on the back of their heads to commemorate Joyce's tattoo and her first day at work without a wig. That kind of positive support is needed in every work environment."

BOLDLY BALD WOMEN

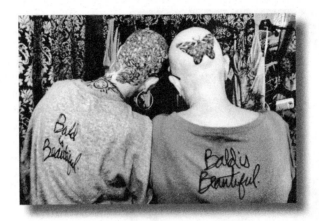

"Joyce and Dotty sporting their Bald is Beautiful
tee-shirts showing off tatooed heads."

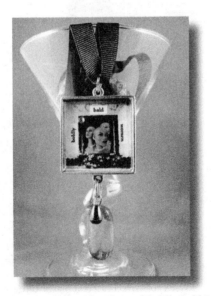

"Joyce and I are working on designs for a line of Boldly Bald Jewelry especially
made for bald women. We have had to suspend this project for a while because
Joyce and Walt's home was destroyed by Hurricane Sandy, and red tape and
reconstruction amid so much devastation for so many will take time. But it will be
worth the wait. Check out our website at www.boldlybaldwomen.com."

BOLDLY BALD WOMEN

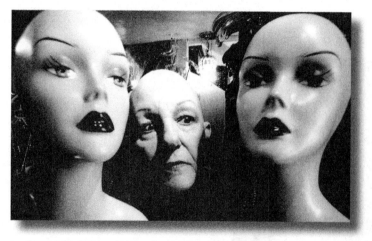

"Wheeeeeresssssss's Waldo, er, I mean Joyce?"

CONTRIBUTORS

𝄞

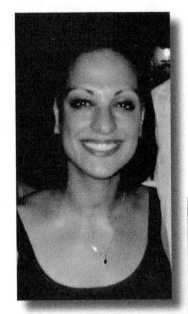

"Caitlin"

"Carol N. Jones"

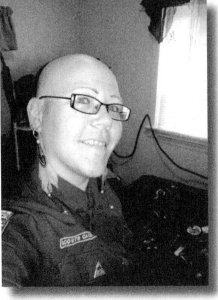

BOLDLY BALD WOMEN

"Carol Solis"

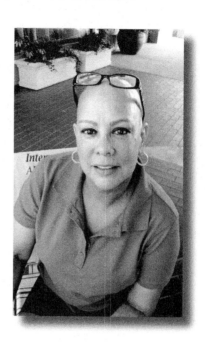

"Dotty and Brett (Scout) Jenkins"

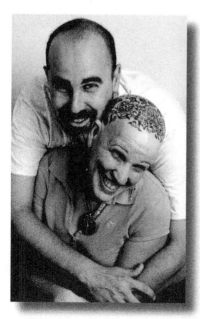

BOLDLY BALD WOMEN

"Faith Reneé Spells"

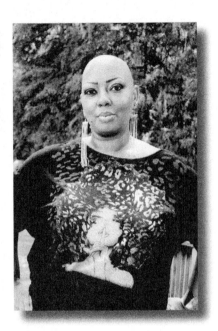

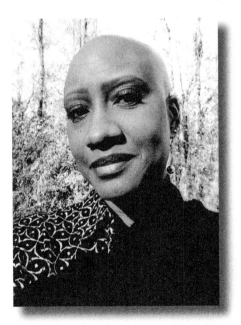

"Galena (Arlene Brooks)"

BOLDLY BALD WOMEN

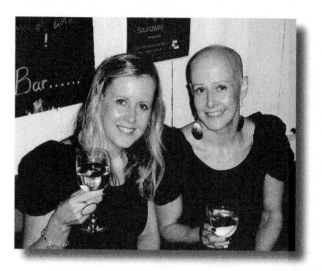

"Gwennan Thomas and her twin sister"

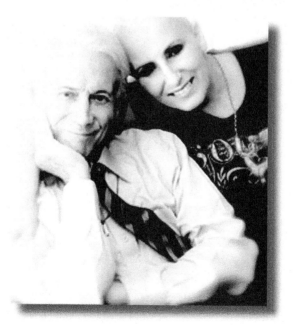

"jO and her father"

BOLDLY BALD WOMEN

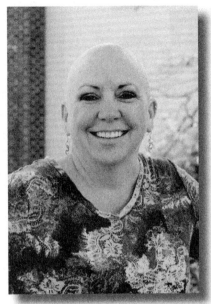

"Karen Denfeld Adams"

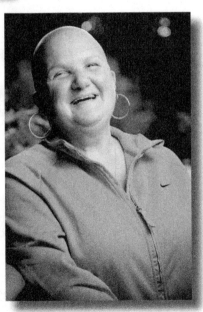

"Kathleen Lyn Rymes,
photo courtesy of Scott Hussey, MSH Marketing Group, Inc."

BOLDLY BALD WOMEN

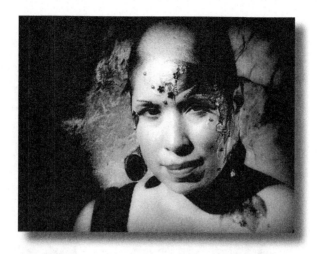

"Kristine Young, photo courtesy of Sarena Mantz, Romantz Photography"

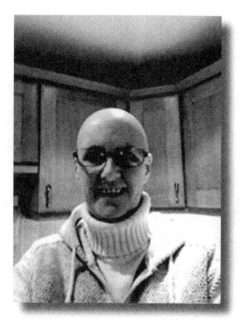

"Margaret Watson"

BOLDLY BALD WOMEN

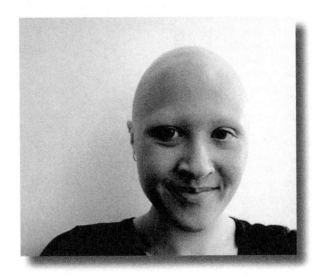

"Megan Sarah Adair"

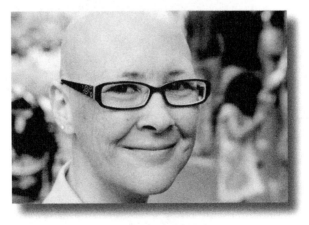

"Sandy Knepp"

BOLDLY BALD WOMEN

"Sarah"

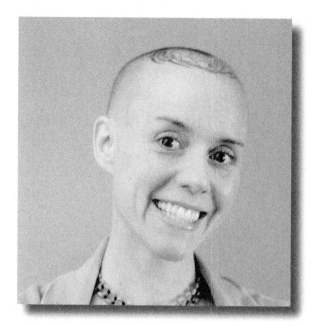

"Sharan Glendinning"

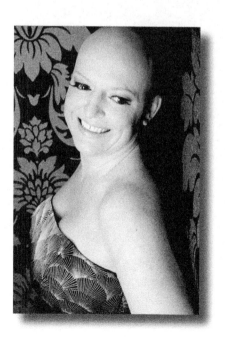

BOLDLY BALD WOMEN

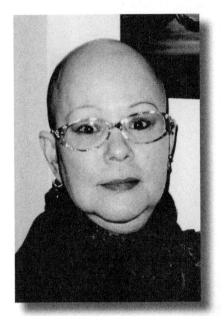

"Willow"

"YoKasta M. Martinez"

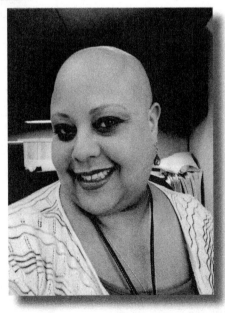

BOLDLY BALD WOMEN

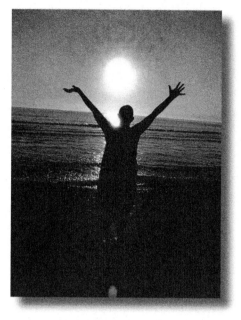

"Joyce"

"I stand for each person suffering in silence...strong, beautiful and full of life. I stand for each girl or boy who couldn't figure out why they were made "different" without hair. I stand for each woman, who after her teens, lost her hair along with her confidence. I stand for myself, having erased the pain, hurt and questions, realizing that my storms weren't for me to seek an umbrella for myself, but to walk in the rain for others."

—Faith Renée Spells

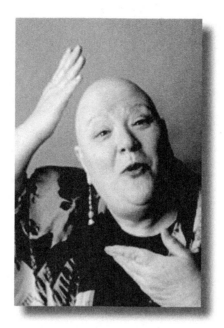

ABOUT THE AUTHOR

Pam lives in Michigan with her husband and their two dogs, Marco Polo and Buddy. She has two adult children and one grand-child. Pam learned to cook Greek cuisine during the ten years she and her husband lived in Athens, Greece, gleaning recipes and techniques from her mother–in–law and sisters–in–law while becoming fluent in Greek. An invitation to a Greek dinner at Mike and Pam's house is rarely ever turned down by family and friends. She is an avid if not always successful gardener. And she is almost learning to enjoy crocheting, thanks to the patient teaching of her expert sister, who says Pam needs a hobby.

Pam has written several children's books for emergent readers based on the Reading Recovery format, and done freelance writing for magazines and business brochures. Pam is available to speak and conduct in-service sessions regarding issues facing bald women in the workplace.

Visit www.boldlybaldwomen.com to become part of the expanding community of boldly bald women and to contact the author.